# YOU'RE NOT A MURDERER: YOU JUST HAVE HARM OCD

Kim Conrey

with

Finn Conrey

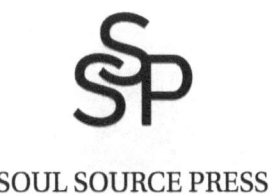

SOUL SOURCE PRESS

An extraordinary aspect of this story is that it is told through both the mother and adolescent's voices, both views written with deep reflection and honesty, as well as infinite love, yearning, and hope. Whether you are working through a similar situation, or you are an adult mentor/educator to families addressing mental illness, or you are interested in knowing more about the realities of family life as the group lives with and through such struggles, you will not be disappointed in this beautiful memoir. I highly recommend *You're Not a Murderer—You Just Have Harm OCD* to you."

—Beverly J. Armento, Author,
*Seeing Eye Girl: A Memoir of Madness, Resilience, and Hope*

This book is dedicated to someone who is curled up on a floor, the corner of a bed, or even nodding at a coworker at the office and pretending they're okay as they wrestle with a panic attack and wonder if their looping thoughts make them a monster.

You are not alone.
You can be free.
This is for you.

# Contents

# FOREWORD

As a psychiatrist for more than 25 years, a Professor of Psychiatry and the Director of Community Psychiatry at Northeast Ohio Medical University, and a member of the Board of Trustees of the Ohio chapter of the National Alliance on Mental Illness (NAMI), I encounter individuals struggling with mental health issues—as well as their beleaguered families—on a regular basis. Something I often notice when talking to those in crisis and their caregivers is how much coded language they've developed with each other to reference the mental condition at the center of their problems without ever explicitly and frankly talking about it.

One of the many things I appreciated about Kim and Finn Conrey's memoir about their individual battles with various forms of obsessive-compulsive disorder (OCD), *You're Not a Murderer: You Just Have Harm OCD*, is how candidly they both document the daily hardships that result from this mental illness. Yet, this book is not a laundry list of woes about how OCD has negatively impacted their lives. Instead, it is a hopeful story about overcoming and creating better lives for themselves through the conscientious practice of exposure and response prevention therapy and, for Finn, finding the psychopharmacological prescription that works best for her.

The authors do not shy away from other difficult, painful subjects, including suicidality. I give suicide prevention talks at the local medical school because the rate of death by suicide among health professionals is even higher than that of the general public. As part of my presentation, I speak to students about the need to have honest dialogs about how they are feeling. At some point during every talk, I will look at the crowd of students and say, "All of you will be around doctors and other clinicians daily the rest of your lives. Shame on you if you cannot ask for help for mental health or substance use issues. You need to help remove the stigma, not promote it. Be honest with each other when a colleague asks how you feel or when someone attempts to tell you how they feel. You have to be willing to have candid discussion about these concerns if you are ever going to help others, the very reason you likely want to be a physician." Therefore, any story written about the mental health journey must contain such honesty if it is to create lasting, real change. You will find such honesty in these pages.

In addition to my other work, I help to coordinate a crisis intervention team (CIT) for first responders, teaching them how to communicate with individuals with mental illness. This weeklong training culminates with the use of role players who act the part of a person in crisis so that police officers and paramedics can practice their enhanced skills of verbal de-escalation. I want them to have empathy and understand that, when called to the residence or other location of a person in a mental health crisis, the family they will encounter there has been dealing with this individual day in and day out for months, years, perhaps decades. This book addresses, with honesty, the exhaustion the family encounters.

The relevance of this to the Conreys' memoir is that they document the process of learning how to verbalize effectively with each other and ultimately provide readers with many good examples of de-escalating communication. Such positive daily encounters, which previously were a major source of stress for everyone involved, help to reinforce that the ways OCD can manifest and present are manageable. This replaces the previous negative cycle with a positive one, in which the person in crisis and the family member both recognize what is happening and short-circuit the disorder's attempt to reinforce itself and its importance to the sufferer. Kim and Finn's documented experiences demonstrate that by depriving OCD of the metaphorical oxygen it needs to promulgate, it loses the ability to control either of their lives.

I am encouraged those individuals in Generation Z, including Finn, are so much more open than previous generations about letting each other know if they are on prescribed medications and/or are receiving mental health assistance. *You're Not a Murderer: You Just Have Harm OCD is a prime example of the kind of candid, thoughtful memoir needed to convince people they are not alone in their mental health struggles and that capable help is available, and often essential.*

—Doug Smith, M.D., DLFAPA
Director of Community Psychiatry
at Northeast Ohio Medical University

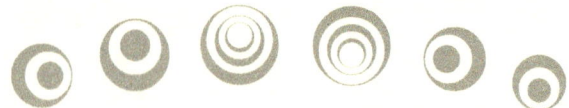

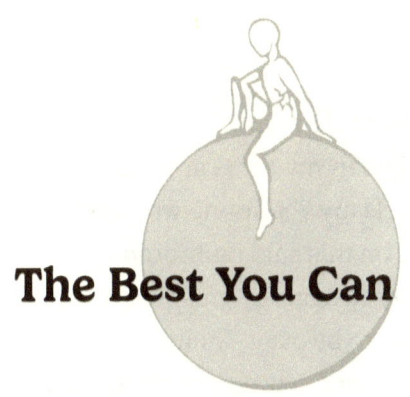

# CHAPTER 1

# The Best You Can

This isn't the first time I've walked into my 18-year-old daughter Finn's room to find her on the bathroom floor crying so hard she can barely breathe, but this time she's dry heaving as well. I'm pretty sure I know why. I'm afraid to ask, afraid to admit to myself that there's a small part of me that doesn't want to ask. A mother's love can't fix this. She isn't a child with a scraped knee. There's no bandage for Harm OCD; images in her head so disturbing that they are as bad as anything from a horror movie. She's the sweetest, most thoughtful human being I've ever met, but she has recurring images of violence: stabbings, shootings, throwing infants down stairs, and the list goes on. To make matters worse, she's the one she sees doing all these horrible things. This is the beast called Harm OCD.

As horrible as it was, it was easier when she just washed her hands until they cracked and bled. I could put ointment on them. There's no ointment for this.

She looks up at me with tears streaming down her face and says, "If all the things I see in my head are true, then I don't deserve to live."

Fear sweeps through my body. My heart pounds and nausea washes over me. It happens every time she says it. We've had this conversation before. Finn assures me she isn't suicidal. Nonetheless, it's a terrifying thing to hear your child say. I get onto the floor of her bathroom with her, a bathroom in dire need of cleaning, which is ironic because of her obsessive-compulsive handwashing. Yet the sink she washes her hands in is filthy. Despite the horrendous nature of OCD, the juxtaposition of those surgically clean hands and filthy sink might bring a small chuckle on any other day.

Not this day.

I wrap my arms around her. At almost 5'11" and 170 pounds, she dwarfs my 5'3" frame when standing, but now she seems so small and frail on this cold bathroom floor. "The things in your head aren't true," I say, struggling, grasping for the right words. "It's just OCD. You're going to be okay. Thoughts are just thoughts, nothing more. This is just a moment in time. It isn't the rest of your life."

"It doesn't feel like it," she says through sobs that shake her body. "I hate this!"

"I know," I say and mean it. At thirteen, I began having similar intrusive thoughts. I was afraid I would intentionally put a pillow over my stepsister's baby and smother him.

In hindsight, I see this for what it was: Harm OCD. I would have never hurt a child. In fact, studies have shown that people with Harm OCD are no more likely to commit violence than the average person, some even show they are less likely to be violent. The empathy and compassion inside the OCD sufferer, and their need to obsessively prove to themselves they would never do such a thing, feeds the beast, intensifying the loop. The more reassurance you give—"Of course, you're a good person. You would never do something like that."—the more it seeks, until one day your heart is racing and stomach is aching, and you cannot cross to the other side of the room without thinking the right thought at the right time. Even if you can hold the right thought in your head, it may morph before you cross the room; then you have to go back, touch a lamp again, or read the same sentence ten times, or as Finn has told me, pick up an eyelash off the carpet because you were thinking about the viciousness of Nazis when you dropped it. If you don't find it, then you're a white supremacist. This is the terrifying, illogical loop OCD can fling us into.

That's the insidious nature of OCD. It wants to get your attention, demands it. It interprets random flashes of nonsense that a neurotypical person would think and say, "Well, that was weird," and move on, as dire warnings. That is why it goes for the most vulnerable thing, the thing that would scare you the most. The thing that is sure to get your attention—and it works. In fact, it works so well that it takes over your mind and then your life. It siphons the joy from moments, steals them, and crushes them. The sufferer will begin to seek confirmation that they are not a murderer, pedophile, or maniac. The sufferer will ask, is this how serial killers start? That's what I thought all those years ago. I now have perspective from the passage of decades and learning about the beast, uncovering its secrets. But, as a teenager, I had never heard the words obsessive-compulsive disorder. So, I sat in a corner of my room whispering, "No, no, no, no." But the more I tried to push OCD away, the more it came for me.

Now, all I can do is hold Finn and assure her she can be free. Last time we visited a therapist, Finn didn't pull back the curtain on the darkest parts of her mind. She must, no matter how painful. Skimming the surface of these dark, churning waters has kept us here. Stuck. Tomorrow, I will contact another therapist . . . and hand Finn a bottle of bathroom cleanser. Seriously, in case you missed it among all the clichés and misunderstanding about OCD sufferers being neat freaks, that's a stereotype. They aren't necessarily clean and orderly.

As I shut the door to her room and head down the stairs to bed, exhaustion sets in deep. I'm a positive person, grateful for opportunities for growth, challenge, transformation, but this . . . I feel stretched thin with holes beginning to form where someone I love might slip through and be lost to me forever . . . Sometimes it's hard to breathe. OCD is a family disease, even if only one person in the home suffers from it. I'm going through a divorce, and I'm sure that isn't helping Finn any. Stress makes OCD worse. I go to bed that night, thinking of all the many ways I failed that day, this year. I add to the guilt list in my head: I forgot to tell my eight-year-old, Brea, to brush her teeth that night. Brea had too much screen time, and I haven't been doing enough speech therapy exercises with her. The worst, though, is that despite all my assurances and all the love in the world, Finn is in absolute torment, and there is nothing I can do. I feel more defeated than I ever have since becoming a mom.

I'm afraid I'm not enough.

Sometime during the night, I dream I'm at my aunt and uncle's home. It is nighttime, and I see my Uncle Richard standing in the backyard as soft light spilling from a window illuminates his face. My aunt still lives there, but my Uncle Richard passed away ten years ago.

He smiles at me and says, "You're doing the best you can in a very difficult situation. It's okay. You're doing a good job."

Despite all the doubt and fear, for one bright moment in the middle of a long, dark night . . .

*I believe.*

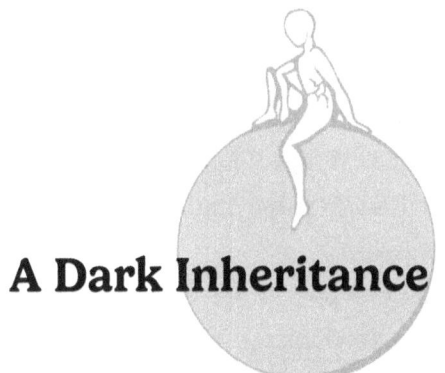

# CHAPTER 2

# A Dark Inheritance

Once, when I was a young girl, my mother sat in the front seat of our Buick and cried as my grandfather stumbled down Bankhead Highway in our small Georgia hometown. In his hand was a liquor bottle wrapped in a brown paper sack. I had never seen him drunk before. I just remembered a sweet old man who wore a fedora and a faded old suit, with circus peanuts and soft peppermint sticks in the pocket of that blazer. We drove away without alerting him we were there. I was too young to know exactly what was happening but old enough to know not to ask about it.

His house was what most nowadays would call a shack. He lived in the old Mill Village—a place where the poorest workers from the cotton mill lived long after it had closed its doors, a relic from the past. That house was home to every stray cat in the neighborhood. He faithfully fed them, and they kept coming. Long divorced, with grandkids only popping in occasionally, he knew more cats than people.

"Here, kitty, kitty. Poor kitty," he would say as he sprinkled food over the ground for the feral horde. I was very young then, but I saw his compassion as he watched the cats pop up one by one about the same time every day, tentatively, slowly, scared. "Poor kitty." He stooped down in well-worn dress shoes, their shine lost long ago from the dust, years, and small-town poverty, to hold out a hand to a cat at once wanting to approach but too frightened at the same time. This was long before rescues were fashionable and the good graces of people like my grandad were where these starving cats turned for help.

Inside the house, you would find no toilet or tub, just an old "slop bucket" and a galvanized washbasin, but you *would* find junk stacked to the ceiling and—I was told—jars of what little money he possessed and other things he considered important hidden in the walls. Perhaps this was some phobia he'd adopted from living through the Great Depression.

His old post office box could be identified immediately by the smudges around the lock. As a little girl, I watched him attempt to leave the post office, get halfway out, perhaps to the parking lot, even almost home, before turning around again to make sure the box was still locked. There was no handle to pull on the small door of the box and confirm it was closed, so he made many attempts to push it with his thumb to make sure it didn't bounce back, which would have showed it was never locked to begin with, as the demanding, panicking part of his brain warned. He'd try to leave again before being steered back by the exhausting compulsion in his brain to check . . . just one more time . . . and again.

As he aged and Parkinson's disease took hold of his limbs, I remember his shaking hand pushing an item on a shelf an inch one way and then the other, and him turning away and then back to do it again. In hindsight, the drinking, and later, a "problem with pills," were clearly signs of a man self-medicating to escape the torment in his head. For me, his kindness was not diminished by what he felt he had to do to survive. I remember a sweet old man communing with feral kindred spirits, moments of peace with feline vagabonds.

Growing up in a Pentecostal family was not the best environment for someone with tendencies toward obsessive-compulsive disorder. For individuals whose brains are wired to feel a sense of foreboding if things aren't done or thought a certain way, the doom of hellfire and brimstone if our lives aren't just so, morally speaking, can trigger an avalanche of intrusive thoughts and compulsions. My oldest sister told me that when she laid in bed at night and heard another family member walking down the hall, she would jump out, get on her knees and pray, and then jump back into bed before they reached the end of the hallway. My mother had intense fears of the devil harming her children.

Motherhood itself can awaken dormant OCD. When Finn was an infant, I began checking the front door incessantly. Finn was a colicky baby who cried for at least an hour or two before finally falling asleep. My husband, Sean and I talked, sang, rocked, and used white noise such as the vacuum cleaner or a running hairdryer draped over a door handle—she wasn't interested in the ocean noise or maternal heart-beat soothing sounds device we had purchased. I think even then she was trying desperately to quiet her mind. I went to bed exhausted, knowing the respite would be short-lived, as she liked to wake up and nurse every couple of hours. But sleep would elude me once the door checking ritual started.

I was twenty-nine then and had managed to escape the dark embrace of OCD since my bout with Harm OCD when I was thirteen. There was the occasional paragraph in a book that I had to go back and reread due to the sense that something terrible would happen—cancer, a car accident, etc.—if I didn't read it again without zoning out. But other than the sporadic blip on the OCD radar screen, I had been keeping it under control. However, having that vulnerable child to protect tripped an alarm in my head that would not be ignored.

One of the first things I noticed about the checking OCD was that it got worse the later I stayed up. If I went to bed when I first became sleepy, I could sometimes bypass the checking ritual. Nonetheless, most moms know that the prime time to get things done is after our children go to sleep. If I went to bed right away, that pile of laundry would not wash itself. Sean did the best he could to help, but he worked the third shift and long hours.

The first instruction most new moms receive is to sleep when the baby sleeps. It is a wonder most mothers don't laugh in the face of those who give such advice. This guidance usually comes from people who are not prepared to show up and clean our houses for us or help our other children with homework while we sleep, or any of the other dozens of things most mothers are taxed with doing.

We live in a society that has no sympathy for exhaustion. We give lip service to the idea of supporting the new mom, but as an older relative quickly told me the first time I mentioned being exhausted after my first child was born, "My mother raised ten kids, and I never heard her complain once." New moms receive about as much support as those with mental health issues— often, little to none. It should come as no surprise that the two are so closely linked, as with postpartum depression. We are a society that likes the sentiment of self-care until we actually catch someone practicing it, then we like to shame them until they get their ass back to work. All mothers know this. This needs to change.

At first, I could get away with checking the door once or twice, but after a couple of weeks, I was checking the door a dozen times or more, the same door, the one I had locked in the first place. Attempts to refuse to go check it again led to a racing heart, sweaty palms, and the abso-lute certainty that my refusal to check for the eighteenth time would result in someone kidnapping or harming my daughter while I slept. OCD showed me barbaric images of my daughter's corpse. This disor-der does not play around, it knows us better than anyone, knows how to get our attention, zeros in on what we hold most dear and scares the hell out of us with that very thing. It held my daughter before me and demanded compliance. This was the penalty for my refusal. I knew this was illogical. But it cannot be stressed enough that OCD does not deal in logic. When the ritual was at its peak, I would begin checking around 10:00 p.m. and finally fall asleep, exhausted, around 2:00 a.m. with nursing Finn and occasionally dozing off in between. One time, as I laid in bed shaking and trying to resist checking *just one more time*, images of my grandfather walking back into the post office over and over again hit me with shocking clarity. *Oh my God. He had OCD.*

Long before Sean and I divorced, I would defer the checking ritual to him.

"Is the door locked?"

"Yes."

"Are you sure?"

"Yes."

"Did you actually try the knob to make sure that it wasn't just barely locked but not really seated in the lock? Sometimes that happens."

"Yep, it's locked."

Sometimes that worked, and sometimes it didn't. He always fell asleep before me. Sometimes I wanted to shake him awake to get him to verify *just one more time* that he'd locked the door. That's the other burden the OCD sufferer carries, guilt. We know we're bothering our loved ones for validation, and we feel bad about it. At the same time, we feel like we're drowning and maybe they'll grab our hand before we sink. Later, we learn they weren't pulling us out; they were pushing us deeper and neither of us realized it. OCD is a clever, insidious disorder.

If I didn't get the validation I could believe before he fell asleep, then it would fall to me to check and recheck. After several weeks of trying to control it on my own without success, I decided I couldn't keep doing this in the same grueling loop. I walked into the library with tears streaming down my face, determined to find a way to help myself. That's when I found a book titled *Brain Lock: Free Yourself from Obsessive Compulsive Behavior*.[1] This book explained the exact mechanisms in the brain that caused OCD.

Detailed explanations appealed to me on many levels. Over the years, I had stopped many a doctor at the door, clipboard in hand, looking to get to his or her next patient, to ask about the specifics of my diagnosis, whether it was a flu, degenerative elbow, or any other issue; I was never content to stop at their diagnosis: I wanted to know where it came from and why it had materialized. This wasn't connected to the

---

1    See endnote 1: Schwartz, Jeffrey, and Beyette, Beverly. (2016). *Brain Lock: Free Yourself from Obsessive-Compulsive Behavior: A Four-Step Self-Treatment Method to Change Your Brain Chemistry*. New York: Harper Perennial

OCD but more a curiosity about the way things work and the need to take responsibility for my health.

*Brain Lock* took that approach and gave the reader credit for being able to understand their OCD. The mindfulness and refocusing the book stressed were helpful for me, and bit by mindful bit, I got my life back. But OCD is never truly cured, and there are still many nights that I look at the front door, feel the urge to check the lock *just one more time*, and have to force myself to walk away. "Just one more time" creates an urge that gets incrementally stronger every time I give in. I know this. There seems to be a window now where I can resist without the cycle starting in earnest, but I know if I give in, if I pull the thread, start the loop . . .

This window of grace wasn't always there. This wasn't always the case. I was just "in." It was sheer torment. Every. Day. I respect the power of OCD and never underestimate the danger of giving in just one more time.

In those dark days, I even played games with my brain where I would picture someone saying, "If your front door is locked, I will give you a million dollars. If not, I will take your house, car, everything." As odd as it may sound, this helped me stop checking the door. I would take "the bet," and eventually this helped me get to sleep. It activated the part of my brain that knew better. After learning more about how the brain works, I suspected that this question bypassed the faulty wiring controlled by OCD—perhaps in the same way that people who stutter when they talk can sing without stumbling over the words. This might also be an example of "the impartial spectator" that Dr. Schwartz refers to in *Brain Lock*.[2] This spectator allowed me to step outside the onslaught and think, apart from the OCD. But it isn't always that easy

---

2   **See endnote 1:** Schwartz, Jeffrey, and Beyette, Beverly. (2016). *Brain Lock: Free Yourself from Obsessive-Compulsive Behavior: A Four-Step Self-Treatment Method to Change Your Brain Chemistry*. New York: Harper Perennial, page 10

and no one solution works for everyone. There are varying degrees of this disorder, bad days and good days.

Just as my grandfather and I had inherited OCD, so had Finn. She never had to have her room "just so" as one might expect from a child with OCD. It was a mess that she was perfectly fine with. There's a huge misunderstanding that people with OCD must have everything neat and orderly. While some sufferers might seek to keep their environment immaculate, this doesn't apply to all of us with OCD; nor does it mean that those who keep their rooms spotless necessarily have OCD. In fact, much to the irritation of those of us who suffer from this crippling neurological disorder, is someone laughing and telling a tidy person, "You're so OCD," or "You're just a germaphobe." It's neither cute nor funny. We don't giggle and tell someone, "You're so Parkinson's," to poke fun at someone who doesn't dance well. Making OCD the punchline of a joke negates the seriousness of the illness. I realize that most people do not understand the torment someone with severe OCD experiences and aren't trying to be hurtful. We've all made comments about things without knowing the seriousness of what we are saying. So, I try to kindly educate when confronted with this situation rather than berate.

Finn's obsessive handwashing started when she was around nine years old. Despite my experiences with OCD, I initially believed the handwashing was simply a reflection of the way schools remind children over and over again about germs and the importance of handwashing. This is great for kids in general, but if you're a mom with a child who has washing OCD, you cringe when your child comes home with a tracing of their hands with little germs drawn in.

Oddly, when it comes to the handwashing, I have realized that Finn and I are opposite sides of the same obsessive coin. While she uses way too much soap and tends to leave soap on her hands making the drying and cracking worse—it's hard to properly rinse that much soap off—I have a fear of leaving any soap on my hands at all. I cringe at the idea of having traces of chemical residue on my skin and rinse for a long time.

I've been in public restrooms, before washing my hands, and started to walk away from the sink when I suddenly get the sensation that there might still be chemicals from the soap on my hands. In the mirror, I notice the lady in line behind me move forward before I put my hands under the faucet to rinse again. I quickly look away so I won't see the strange look on her face that I'm certain must be there. I've had to force myself to leave the sink when people are waiting in line. My heart pounds harder as I walk away. Now that I'm older, I'm able to let it go. That wasn't always the case.

"Stop using so much soap," I pleaded with Finn. "You only need a drop or two and rinse them a little better. Don't leave any soap. That will dry your hands out." I didn't realize it at the time, but she was washing them quickly to complete the ritual and having lots of soap was more important to her ritual than rinsing it all off. Despite my soap issues, Sean was an impartial judge that determined she was going through bottles of hand soap quicker than we could get to the store to buy them.

"I like the foamy stuff," she said.

"Yeah, me too. But you're tearing up your skin."

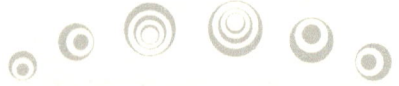

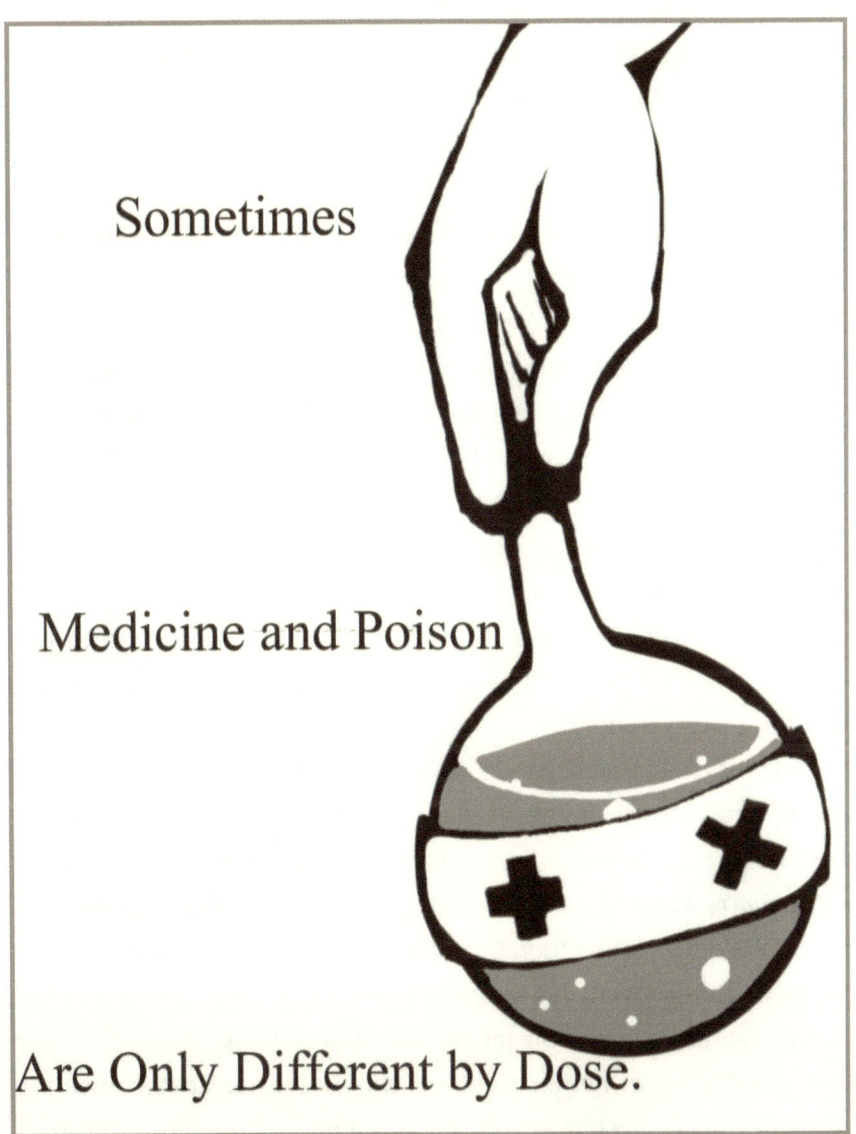

Sometimes

Medicine and Poison

Are Only Different by Dose.

**Illustration by Finn Conrey**

Over the next year, her hands felt like sandpaper, and they began cracking. When I rubbed lotion on them, it seeped into the dry fissures, and she jerked her hands away and tears sprang to her eyes as she told me the lotion made them sting worse.

"You have to stop this, Finn. God made dirt, and dirt doesn't hurt. Your immune system will appreciate a little dirt. Look at it that way."

"At school, they tell us to wash our hands after going to the bathroom and before eating."

"Just stop using so much soap. It isn't necessary."

I hoped the handwashing was just a phase, not the initial symptom of a much larger problem, but she soon began coming home and telling me that her friends needed her to keep them out of trouble. And she could tell her vigilance was irritating them.

"Well, is it something that could cause harm to them or yourself?"

"Not always. It's just that they aren't thinking."

"Maybe you could let it go if no one is going to get hurt. Sometimes kids do goofy things, and if no one is in danger, then maybe you just shouldn't worry about it."

Looking back, I realize that "just shouldn't worry about it" is suitable advice for most children, but when someone with OCD hears this, the beast lurking in their mind sounds an alarm: *It's a trap—telling me not to worry means I should worry even more.* And the OCD doubles down. We didn't know then that reassuring her was actually making things worse—so were our expectations.

Finn has always been the tallest person in her class. When I saw her in single file line at her elementary school, she was always towering above her peers, even the boys. There is a natural tendency to expect more from taller children. We don't even realize we're doing it. They also accepted her into the gifted program early on. For someone who already felt the weight of the world from OCD, this all culminated in creating the perfect storm.

## Finn says:

I remember my first experience with Harm OCD. I was in elementary school, and the group of friends I was with were going just a foot outside the boundary on the playground. I began panicking. It wasn't a big deal. They could still be clearly seen, but I remember being hit by this intense fear, thinking we shouldn't be doing this. We could all be in trouble, kidnapped, or killed by bad people because we didn't listen! And that was all I could think of. Images of carnage flooded my mind on a loop. So, I went and told the teacher despite my friends' protests. After that, I went about my day as best as I could, in my mind having just averted disaster for my friends and me.

This continued all throughout my time in elementary, middle, and high school. I always felt like there was something off about me. I worried far more than any of the other kids, and I knew that even to my friends, I could be an annoying goody-goody, a worrywart, a killjoy, a snitch. My parents and my teachers assured me I was just mature for my age, that this pressure to look after all of my friends and be responsible for their wellbeing was a good thing. Little did they know they were enabling my invasive thoughts and the "validity" of those thoughts, causing me to listen to them more. I always felt like I wasn't able to do what I wanted. I had to care for other people first and because of that, I felt as though I had grown up really fast.

Looking back on it now, I realize it was OCD, and all of the praise that I received for being so "responsible" just fed the beast and made me keep worrying about it. The intrusive thoughts I was having about bad things happening to my friends were not normal worries, as I had been led to believe. It is not the fault of those who did praise me for being worried, though. They couldn't have known this wasn't regular worry. They thought they were making me feel good about being responsible. And while it is nice to create responsible kids, I began to think it was the only thing I was good for.

I didn't realize all of this at the time though. It was a slow and creeping thing that took years to fully develop, and each little instance was kindling for a flame that turned into an inferno.

# The Weight of the World

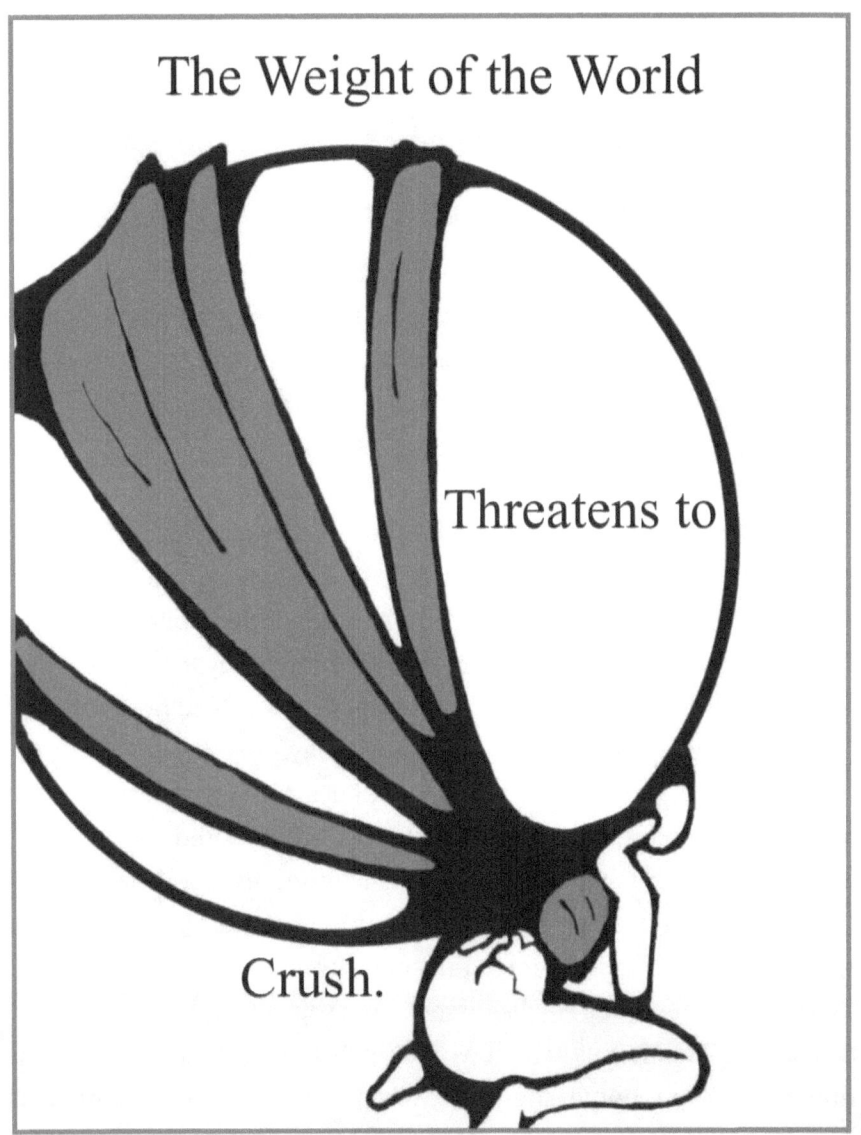

Threatens to

Crush.

Illustration by Finn Conrey

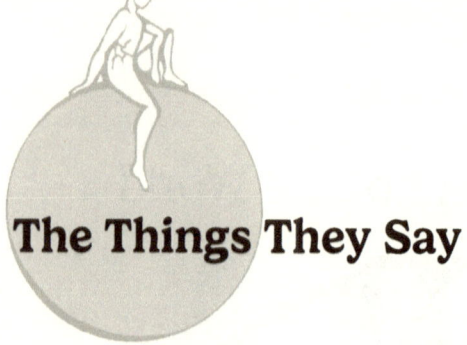

# CHAPTER 3

# The Things They Say

Finn had a thoughtful look on her face as I cleared empty cups and cracker crumbs from the kitchen table. The neighbor's grandkids had just gone home from a playdate with her. Our little ranch houses sat side by side with their grandmother's, and Finn would look out the window, just waiting for them to visit.

"Why don't I have a brother or sister?" she asked.

"Well, we were busy having fun with you, and now your dad is away in Afghanistan." I didn't really want to tell her that Sean and I had been having issues on and off for years, and having another child was a step too far. He and I were barely more than roommates by that point.

"But a brother or sister is a forever friend." Tears filled her eyes.

"I know, sweetie. I'm sorry. Maybe someday."

While Sean was away, Finn developed a fever that lasted for a few days. Afterwards, she broke out in hives that coated her body. At one point, the only place I could locate without hives was her nose. I couldn't trace it to any allergy or a reaction to something new in her environment. When we went to the doctor, there were only one or two tiny hives on her torso. He dismissed it as a slight allergic reaction and advised antihistamines, which we'd already tried with no success. An hour after we got home, she was covered head to toe once more. For almost four days, she clawed and cried.

"I can't stand it. Why won't they stop?"

All I could find online was a reference to viral-induced hives.

On the third night, when the hives were at their worst, I begged her to just sit on her hands to stop scratching. She clawed them so much her skin was starting to bleed. It was the first time since I'd become a mom that I had experienced what it was like to have no answers. After she fell asleep, I knelt beside her bed and begged God to take them away. I loathed not having the answers, the cure, the ability to make it all right. I hoped to never feel that kind of parental helplessness again. I had no idea how much worse that feeling could get, but I was about to find out.

My marriage took a turn for the better after Sean returned from serving overseas and resumed his job as an aircraft technician. It seems we'd both needed time apart to gain some perspective. We tried to give Finn a sibling. During 2011 and 2012, when Finn was around 10 years old, I lost two pregnancies. It was a hope and devastation roller-coaster ride.

I was happy to learn I was pregnant in 2011 but then began experiencing symptoms of miscarriage. I would go to the doctor's office crying and accepting that no one could bleed that much and still be pregnant, and yet, when I went in for an eight-week ultrasound, the technician said the heartbeat was great and that I was only six weeks along.

"I know I'm eight weeks along," I told my doctor.

"Oh, that's okay. People miscalculate all the time."

I knew I hadn't. Something was wrong, but she continued to reassure.

"Congratulations. This is a viable pregnancy. Sometimes people have scary symptoms but still carry to term. The heartbeat is strong," my doctor assured me.

I went home hopeful but worried. The bleeding would stop for a few days then begin again. Hope and devastation followed each other in a loop, wearing me down.

As I closed in on the end of the first trimester, the spotting got worse yet again. We went back for another ultrasound, and this time there was no telltale flashing on the screen. My palms began to sweat. The technician said nothing for several moments as she searched at different angles to confirm what the lump in my throat and my shallow breathing already knew. The heartbeat had stopped.

The ride home was quiet. I bled on and off over the weekend as we took Finn to the movies and went about our lives. Then Sunday night I woke with searing, icy cold lower-back pain that came in waves all night long.

I felt like Sean wasn't taking my grief seriously enough. He and I fought periodically all weekend, but we tried our best not to do it around Finn. I'd still not been able to figure out how to tell her. Or perhaps I was procrastinating—or both.

That Monday morning after dropping Finn off at school, we sat in silence at the kitchen table with our mugs of coffee. *What the hell does it matter if I have the caffeine now?* "Does the miscarriage bother you, too?" I asked him.

"Well, honestly, and don't get mad at me for saying this, but I don't feel the same connection with it that you do."

I nodded. "Yeah, I get it." And I did, but the answer made me feel completely alone. From the start, she was with me, beneath my heart, always. He would never experience it the same way, which wasn't his fault.

He came inside from doing yardwork around noon and asked me to help him flip the mattress. "It hasn't been flipped in a while." He liked to flip it every six months.

I wanted to cuss, scream, or throw something. I didn't want to flip a mattress while life drained from my body. But I didn't say anything. I helped flip the mattress, stewed for a while, then walked outside to tell him how hurt I was. We argued back and forth again. It's now a haze of grief and hurt feelings that I no longer remember in detail. The whole incident ended with him going to get me my favorite sandwich for lunch. Sometimes people don't know what to say. Sometimes they can only *do*.

Later that day, when Finn came home from school, I told her the baby was gone, and that we could try again. I kept my tone upbeat and hopeful, believing I was doing the best thing for her, but the next day she went to school and cried at her desk until a teacher asked her what was wrong. She told them she had lost her brother or sister. I hadn't shown her any of my emotions, and now she felt like she wasn't entitled to them either. I failed her again.

I grieved more than I thought possible, astounded that I could have become so close to a child I'd never met. I searched the internet, looking for reassurance that having a second miscarriage was a fluke, and I found plenty. The odds of having two losses in a row were only two percent.

A couple months later, I became pregnant again, and two ultrasounds revealed a robust heartbeat. But I started bleeding again, and both ultrasounds revealed a discrepancy between when I knew I'd conceived and the date the ultrasound technician estimated from what she was seeing.

"Hey, some women just bleed when they are pregnant. It doesn't necessarily mean you'll miscarry. The heartbeat is still strong," my doctor told me.

But in my soul, I'd already begun grieving. The night before, I dreamed of a choir singing in some other realm, and I noticed one of them holding a baby wrapped in a blanket. *She'll never make it here.*

We took Finn to Saint Augustine to visit the beach for a few days. One of my favorite spots in the world is the shrine of Nuestra Senora de la Leche y Buen Parto on the grounds of the Catholic church downtown, Nombre de Dios. The first mass on North America was held on that very spot when Pedro Menendez's fleet landed there in 1565. The grounds are lush green with a pond out front, filling and draining with the tides and exposing the unlikely, tiny crabs with one giant claw and one small one. They scuttle into their holes as visitors approach. A trail passes through the grounds, taking us past a 208-foot steel cross, a giant statue of the chaplain of Menendez's fleet, Fr. Francisco Lopez de Mendoza, graves of nuns that taught freed slaves to read in the 1880s, and several other alcoves with small shrines and ongoing archeological digs.

The church reports getting hundreds of letters from all around the world from women asking them to say a prayer at the shrine for a safe birth. Even though my view of spirituality had evolved over the years to a decidedly more ecumenical one as I read works by the Dalai Lama, Henry David Thoreau, Wayne Dyer, Dan Millman, and others, I was fully prepared to go beg the God of my youth to save my baby.

I headed to the small chapel, first built in the late 1600s but rebuilt many times following hurricanes and the toll of time. I walked into the ivy-covered, open-air, stifling-hot little sanctuary, where I lit a candle, made the sign of the cross, and kneeled to pray. The smell of candle wax mingles with the salty breeze coming in the small windows from the Matanzas River. The candles burn constantly, regardless of how hot and humid it is outside. Devotion need not be comfortable.

In front of me is a statue of Mary nursing the Christ child. I prayed, bargained, and pleaded for my baby to make it this time. I prayed Finn would find relief from her anxiety, and then I got up and committed to spend the rest of the weekend trying not to let my own anxiety keep me from enjoying time with my family.

We spent the next few days in the waves with Finn. On the ride home, I wondered over and over again whether the baby's heart was still beating. During times of high stress, the OCD can come back disguised as an old friend intending to help me. Luckily, I knew better. At a rest stop halfway between the beach and home, I felt my leg brush against the seat in an odd way as I exited the car. I had a thought flash through my mind that if I could get back in the car and back out again without my leg brushing the seat, my baby would make it this time.

*Oh, no you don't!*

*But wouldn't you do it to save your baby?*

The logical side of my brain knew this brand of nonsense and didn't give in. However, my heart began beating faster, and I felt panic surge through me. Yet I kept walking, absolutely sure that one step back toward the car to repeat the action, one step in that direction, always equaled ten.

A few days later, Sean and I pulled into the parking lot of the OB/GYN, and the first thing I saw when I opened the door was a dead bird lying on the asphalt. *Don't go there. It doesn't mean anything.* Sean walked up beside me. I pointed to the ground. "That's a bad sign."

"Nope. It's just a dead bird. Happens all the time."

*Miscarriages happen all the time. I'm supposed to be okay with that.*

We sat in the waiting room, anticipating and dreading our turn with the ultrasound technician. I felt nauseous. The room was too cold. A couple walked out smiling and laughing while looking at a little picture.

"Congratulations," I said as they sat down beside my husband and me.

"Thank you!" they each said as they waited on the nurse to return with their paperwork.

I felt a sliver of anger creep in that they might never know how hard it would be to wait on what I was sure would be more bad news. A good person would never want someone else to feel this way, I thought. I also said a prayer that I knew some might find cold. *God, if this baby isn't going to make it, then please let this already be over when I go in there.* I couldn't take a third ultrasound with another strong heartbeat only to have to go home and wait for the inevitable. At that point, the hope was hurting me more than the devastation could. These days of bleeding followed by days of nothing and assurances of strong heartbeats only to be followed by more signs of miscarriage were wearing me down.

At last, the nurse called my name. *You're going to be okay either way.* Walking into the darkened room, I spotted the hulking piece of machinery that would deliver the verdict; it would be devastating either way because I knew a heartbeat didn't always mean we would stay pregnant. Sean seemed nervous as well but said little.

I couldn't bear the pleasant banter with the technician. So, as I lay down on the crinkling paper, I told her how we'd lost the last baby and that I was having miscarriage symptoms with this one as well. I wanted to protect the technician, too: if she smiled and perhaps asked us what gender we were hoping for, she would feel bad when she had to deliver terrible news to us.

The bright flashing light and thumping heartbeat that had reverberated off the walls of the darkened room mere weeks earlier were now replaced by inescapable silence. And then sobs from me and apologies from the technician. At twelve weeks, this heartbeat had stopped as well. I felt I had failed my baby and Finn, again. I wondered if her heartbeat had gone silent as I stood in the Atlantic with the waves washing over me, receding, and coming back again, taking her soul back to the other side to begin again. Somehow, if she had to go away, that felt right to me.

On the car ride home, I texted my best friend, Cherie, with the news. She had been hoping, praying, and encouraging every step of the way. I wished I had better news for both of us. She sent back condolences.

At least this time I didn't have to worry about Finn. I had decided not to tell her at all until we were well out of the woods. Not only didn't we make it out of the woods, but I was also well and truly lost deep inside them. I decided I didn't want to spend several days cramping and waiting for the inevitable again. This time I asked the doctor to do a procedure where the baby could be removed and sent for testing. Maybe there was some answer, some reason why this was happening. Luckily, Finn had been invited to a sleepover that night after school. So, I was able to go to the outpatient facility and then rest that night without Finn knowing about any of it.

As we pulled up to the outpatient surgical building for the appointment, Sean and I fought again. All these years later, I can't recall what the argument was about. I only remember deep sorrow and grief, dumping words and emotions into a gulf that could not be filled. We sat in the car verbally tearing into each other. I cried as I got out of the car, checked in, and walked down the hallway to the operating room.

I woke up in post op with other patients in various stages of coherence. I heard a woman sobbing and recognized a second later that it was me. A nurse rushed over. Her hand found its way to mine beneath the blanket.

"I'm sorry," I kept repeating, embarrassed that I was crying so hard, worried that I was burdening her with my emotions. "I can't breathe."

"You're hyperventilating. Concentrate on long, slow breaths." She leaned over to whisper so that only the two of us could hear: "I lost a baby, too. It hurts. I'm *so* sorry."

Finally, someone said it. Her words were simple. They were profound. Somewhere inside I felt my soul sigh in relief and settle for the first time in a long while. Breathing came easier. The nurse brushed the hair back from my face as I read her name tag over and over again: *Melissa*. I was determined to remember her name so I could thank her later.

Grief cut deep and jagged, but gratitude trailed healing from her wings as she gently passed by.

A week later, I brought a card into the outpatient center and dropped it off at the nurse's station. I thought she might read it, smile, and move on. Later that day, I was shocked when she called to thank me. She told me how nursing was her calling and how much it meant to her. Even in the darkest of nights, there is someone holding a lamp.

From all the mothers I've asked about this, I have learned that everyone is different. Not everyone will understand. Not everyone has to. Some mothers say it isn't a big deal; some take years to move on. Any of these reactions are valid for that person, at that moment in time.

But as for me, I spent a solid three months carrying this person beneath my heart. When I walked into the outpatient surgical building, even though her heart wasn't beating, she was still with me. When I woke, I knew she was gone. No, I never held her or knew her personality, but in my mind, we'd played together, I'd seen her in the backyard with her sister, I'd held her while she slept as I felt her warm breath on my neck.

Later that evening, as I lay across the bed, drifting in and out of sleep, I heard the bedroom door creak open. Sean placed his hand on my back and left it there a second. I assumed he was checking to see if I was still breathing.

I didn't say anything, but I noticed, and it mattered.

Finally, we became pregnant again. Though some of the closeness Sean and I had gained as a couple after his return from Afghanistan had waned, we still wanted to give Finn a sibling and we cared about each other. But as the pregnancy progressed, I couldn't relax. I held my breath through every ultrasound, and I had many of them, as I was 39 by that time and had already experienced two losses. I later learned that the long-drawn-out miscarriages, where the fetus grows slowly but maintains a heartbeat—at least for a while—tended to point to a trisomy pregnancy, which is common in older mothers. The eggs grow "sticky" with time and often hold on to the extra set of chromosomes that are supposed to "spin away" when the cells replicate. The trisomy most people are familiar with is Down Syndrome, because this is one of the few trisomies that can survive outside the womb. My doctor had sent our last miscarriage to the lab and determined that our second loss was a trisomy-10, which is nearly always fatal.

After a very stressful pregnancy of high-risk specialists and a dangerous condition called preeclampsia—characterized by severely high blood pressure and stress to the kidneys and liver—we had another baby girl. I'd even let Finn name her. A little boy in her martial arts class was named Bregan. I told her I liked the name. She thought for a moment and said, "Breaganna." I loved it immediately. Though it's rarely pronounced right, I can't blame anyone for that.

But our joy soon turned to grief as Finn missed spending time with me. As an only child for eleven years, she had grown accustomed to having me all to herself—learning to share me with her new sister was difficult for her. I did all I could to carve out time for them both, but exhaustion and lack of sleep left me feeling depleted.

"Please don't go," Finn would beg. She held on to my arm as Brea wailed in the other room.

"I'm sorry. She is in there crying, and I can't ignore her. I love you. I'll be back." I never dreamed how much it would tear me in half to have another child or what could be worse than that.

I was soon to find out.

One Sunday afternoon when Breaganna was about five months old, I walked into the room where I'd left Finn playing a computer game while Brea slept on the bed beside her. I found Finn in tears. "What's wrong, honey?"

"I keep thinking about killing Brea," she sobbed out. "I had my hand on her neck when I thought it. I wasn't choking her. It was just . . . there. Maybe I was going to kill her."

I sat down on the bed beside them, and my heart started pounding wildly as I watched Brea sleeping peacefully.

I called Sean into the room. "We need your help in here."

"I can't. I need to go clear the weeds from the sewage line in the front yard. They're backed up again."

Every few years, roots would grow across the sewage access pipe to the house, and if we did not clear it in time, sewage would back up into the house.

"I don't care. Do it later," I said. I didn't want to be left alone with this. I explained what was happening, and he did his best to reassure her.

"It's just a random thought. We all get flashes of nonsense. It's meaningless. Let it go."

"I can't!" she wailed.

He turned his head at the sound of gurgling coming from the hall bathroom. "I've got to go."

"Oh, you mean it's backing up right now?"

"Yup." He turned and sprinted down the hallway for old towels and then out the door to dig the roots out of the pipe.

It seemed fate, the Universe, God, or however one chooses to see it, felt that it was my challenge to work through. *Of course, it was.* Years ago, I knew a pastor that used to say, "First in the natural and then in the spiritual." He felt that situations manifested in the natural realm first. Then later, one would see what was to come in the spiritual, or in this instance, the mental. If that's the case, then weed roots growing across a channel that's made to carry sewage away from a home is an absolute perfect metaphor for intrusive thoughts backing up inside someone's head instead of being carried away as the nonsense, detritus, crap thoughts that they truly are in a neurotypical brain. The fact that it happened at precisely that moment has always seemed oddly appropriate or perfectly synchronous.

"How do you know I won't kill her?" she asked.

"Because I had those same thoughts about my stepsister's baby when I was a kid, and I never hurt him, and you won't hurt her either. It's a random thought. We attach too much meaning to it. The thoughts often came when I was holding him or playing with him. It was just a random flash the first time, but then I tried not to think about it, and that seemed to start a loop." Once more I remembered the horror of the images that had run over and over again in my head: I saw myself holding a pillow against his face. It terrified me to my core. The more I pushed the thoughts away, the worse they got.

"But how do you know I won't do it?"

And there it was, the scrupulous devotion to certainty that OCD demands but can never achieve, because "for sure," "never," and "forever" are impossible conditions. No one can ever truly guarantee something. We can only be content with knowing who we are. It must be enough, but it will never be enough for the demanding beast called OCD. It's also a beast that traps. How in the world does the person with OCD, especially Harm OCD, tell someone that they've pictured themselves killing them, and, worse, that the violent images are playing on a sickening loop?

I didn't tell her that I'd had another flare up of Harm OCD after watching *Silence of the Lambs* when I was eighteen. On the drive home from the theater, I couldn't stop thinking about the movie. I quizzed my boyfriend over and over again about whether I was a menace to society, trying to drag reassurances out of him.

"What if I'm a murderer, and I just don't know it yet?"

"You aren't. Don't worry about it. You're a good person."

"Tell me you know for sure I would never do anything like that."

"You won't do anything like that!" He was sympathetic but also seemed baffled by my sudden demanding questions that made no sense to him. He was an engineer with a knack for logic and solid connections. OCD cares nothing for the frail vagaries of logic. It believes there is some deeper, absolute truth, and if it just keeps digging, it will find it.

It won't.

I asked him, "But how can you know for sure?"

"I don't know. I just do."

The dark road blurred before me as I remembered my first bout with Harm OCD. Though just like then, I had no idea it was OCD, much less being able to specify that it was Harm OCD.

"When you were a kid, were you ever afraid you would kill one of your siblings?"

"Yes. It crossed my mind, but it doesn't mean anything."

This made me feel a little better. But I didn't drop it there. It haunted me for another few months before fading. *Taking someone with Harm OCD to a horror film pretreatment isn't the best idea.*

The reason I didn't tell Finn about the movie trigger was because the last thing I wanted was to plant that seed in her head. She might start avoiding all forms of entertainment for fear of getting triggered.

Now I watched my child deal with this. I had hoped since she grew up in a more stable home, she wouldn't have this problem. I often thought that my fight with OCD had to do with living in homes with violent people. My mother came from a charismatic church that encouraged parents to whip children as much and as long as it took—and she did. My stepmother was worse, flying into rages with little to no warning. She would scream, hit, and throw things. But in the nature versus nurture realm, OCD tended to surface regardless of circumstance, though anxiety can worsen it, for sure. All these things crossed my mind as Finn sobbed and shook while Breaganna slept, and my heart broke.

She said, "I'm supposed to be the hero, like in my video games. But I'm the villain. I can't be the villain. Those are terrible people!"

"Every hero has a tragic backstory," I told her. Even though she was only eleven, we'd discussed the heroes in her books and games and how their "backstory" influenced who they became. "They all had something to overcome. This is yours. And it's okay."

"No, it isn't."

She collapsed in my arms as I felt my world tilt and shatter. I was angry that she should have to deal with this instead of enjoying being a kid. But OCD doesn't care. "You're still a baby yourself," I said as I smoothed her long, wavy hair back to reveal tears trailing down her face. "I know who you are. I'm your mother. You won't hurt her."

"But *how* do you know?" she pleaded.

"Because I know *you*."

Later that evening as she watched SpongeBob, she burst into tears again. The world of cartoons, giggling, and innocence had been slashed by the sharp talons of OCD. I became angry at myself. Maybe I could have taken a certain vitamin while I was pregnant or been less stressed out when she was little. Like most mothers, I searched for answers in futility, and I turned the blame inward.

"You can't change it, Finn," her dad said. "All you can do is move forward."

Nothing we said that day or any day after was enough.

I lay in bed that night next to Sean feeling hopeless. "I wish I could turn the clock back to a few days ago before all this happened."

"I do, too," he said. "She'll be fine. It's just a thought. She didn't hurt Brea."

"I know." I remembered the first time OCD had roared in my face. It stamped my life with a sorrow that could never be undone. I knew we'd just crossed a dividing line from which our lives could not rewind, and Finn would never be the same. As bad as that day was, I hadn't even begun to understand what the next decade would bring.

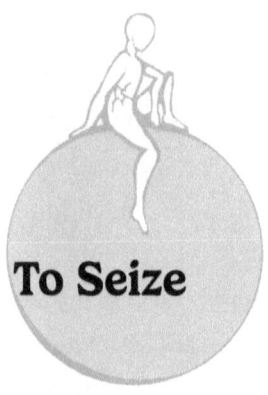

# CHAPTER 4

# To Seize

I took care of Brea and Finn under a cloud of silence and worry. I assured myself that Finn's recent confession was no different from when I was thirteen and had the intrusive thoughts of Harm OCD, and I turned out okay. But there was one big difference: now I was the mother hearing these horrible things. I never spoke to my mother about it. Though I became Catholic when I married Sean, I grew up in a charismatic Christian church that believed demons were responsible for everything from losing one's car keys to a couple getting divorced. Telling her about my intrusive thoughts would've meant the endless humiliation of an exorcism as every elder in the church attempted to be a hero and pray the demon out of me. I knew first-hand that this could happen.

My mind drifted back in time to an old white church building with windows frosted to make sure you couldn't see out and get distracted— the real world, a distorted blur. The building smelled perpetually of spearmint gum and a slight mold that drifted from the basement. These odors lingered in my nostrils when I was around nine years old and battling some sort of stomach bug. I felt sick and attempted to sit down during the long song service that preceded the sermon, but my grandmother gave me "the look," so I stood back up. I knew she would tell my mother, and I would get in trouble if I sat down. Yellow spots clouded my vision before everything went dark. I passed out and hit my head on the back of the pew and then fell to the tile floor, where I hit my head again. As soon as I came to, I saw the puffy feet of old church matriarchs sticking out of their well-worn pumps like bloated leaches.

"Is 'er eyes dilated?" I heard one of the matriarchs ask as she smacked her gum.

This was followed by the voice of our pastor asking that I be brought to the pulpit. My grandmother marched me to the front where the pastor waited. The back of my dress felt cold and damp against my legs. I realized I had wet myself when I fainted. One humiliation stacked upon another.

He slapped a clammy hand against my bruised forehead and proclaimed, "Satan! You will not use this child to interrupt this service!"

Nine-year-olds don't have everything figured out, but I knew I had a stomachache, not a demon. What would happen in such a church if someone told another parishioner, or God forbid *that* pastor that they were having the looping, violent thoughts of Harm OCD? If a demon is responsible for everything from divorce to lost car keys, then what in the world would such a church do with intrusive thoughts?

A few years before that, during a moment of prayer after a particularly hysterical sermon about hell, the devil, and his various legion of minions, the pastor told us to search our hearts. I closed my eyes and thought about God but didn't see anyone attempting to throw me into hell. Instead, a soft light coalesced in my mind. It radiated acceptance, contentment, joy, and formed a type of face that smiled at me. I smiled back as tears ran down my face. It knew me. I knew it. We've been good ever since.

However, I'm fairly certain what the consequences would have been amongst the parishioners, not God, had I admitted to unbidden thoughts of smothering a child. A treatable neurological disorder would not have been the first assumption of anyone in that congregation. I can only imagine how many people throughout the ages—kind, gentle souls—have been demonized, banished, and likely even burned at the stake or received some other horrific fate for confiding in someone about this disorder.

My older sister had epilepsy, but she wasn't told the reason for the facial contortions she was experiencing and the moments of lost time due to absence seizures or the grand mal seizure that had her waking up in the hospital. She would later tell me she had stood in front of the mirror saying, "Stop it! Stop it!" as she tried to control her facial movements. She confessed she'd been afraid she was losing her mind. The reason no one had discussed the word "epilepsy" with her was that they were afraid she would tell someone.

The term epilepsy was a dangerous word to use in a Pentecostal church. A demon-possessed man in the Bible was referred to as being an "epileptic." Of course, this word means "to seize." And though Hippocrates had tried to tell everyone that he thought it was due to a disorder in the brain, the vast majority of the last 2,300 years has seen people coming up with more colorful and damaging theories to explain this phenomenon. My parents wouldn't tell my sister it was epilepsy because they feared people would assume a demon possessed her if she used that word. And God help her if they thought that!

I was having none of that nonsense when it came to my own child. OCD, no matter how frightening, or what kind of intrusive thoughts may come with it, is a neurological disorder. However, I have to admit to being too afraid initially to seek help. I feared that, even though most trained psychologists would know better, they would believe her capable of hurting Brea, and I might lose one of them to a foster home due to a well-meaning therapist demanding they be separated.

After having taken Finn to several mental health professionals, I now know that they don't think this way. They understand and have told me that there isn't any danger from Finn. They've also shared with both me and Finn that all the things she has experienced are typical for people suffering with Harm OCD. But I didn't know that back then. We all do our best with what we understand, and although a group of Pentecostal elders trying to pray demons out of a frightened child seems beyond ridiculous to me now, they were working within a framework they understood. Now we know better. There is no further excuse.

Christmas was a week away. We decorated the house with a big tree in the living room, garland and lights draped over the mantle. I hoped the holidays would bring some joy and respite from Finn's worries. She and I sat at the kitchen table eating our lunch while Brea took her nap. I was sad to know that while most children were obsessing over their presents, Finn was obsessing over whether she was a murderer, despite all my assurances that she wasn't. When I looked back over her childhood, I saw a pattern of excessive worry. She was only eleven years old, but she already carried more emotional weight than most adults I knew.

Years later, she would tell me about having to scratch her legs or arms in an even pattern. "If I scratched my left leg, I'd have to scratch my right leg, but I might accidentally scratch it in a slightly different place, which meant I'd have to go back and scratch the other one to make it even. But, uh oh, I might have scratched one harder than the other, so I'd have to go back and scratch the first one with the same intensity, even though it no longer itched. I knew it didn't make any sense, and I would try to stop, but then I would start to panic."

I especially hated tying her shoes for her. She would obsess over one being tighter than the other. We would untie and retie the one she said was too loose, but then she would say the other one wasn't right. We would loosen or tighten the other, only to find that it was out of balance with the other once more. Her father and I would eventually get exhausted with it and tell her to just live with it. This would often cause her to either break down in tears or get angry and stomp her feet. Even children without OCD can have things they like a certain way, so we didn't jump straight to an OCD explanation.

I recalled a few Christmases earlier when Finn looked up from opening a present, burst into tears, and said, "I don't want to die!"

Not long before that incident, our cat had gotten out of the house and was hit by a car. This began an avalanche of questions about death. I was hoping for something to soothe her mind. Of course, we told her what our faith taught about the afterlife. We even discussed the idea of reincarnation. She watched an animated series where one character was a reincarnation in a long line of monks with elemental powers. We checked out books meant to explain the concept of death to children, but they were vague with analogies about trees returning in the spring. She wanted to know the details. She wanted concrete assurances: the kind OCD demands.

I asked other parents if they went through this with their kids. While a friend of mine and I waited for our kids outside our church, I told her about Finn randomly bursting into tears. I recounted the painful questions she asked about death: "What if I die first and you aren't in heaven, and I'm scared?" "What if I reincarnate to another family and never find you again?" How could anyone answer such questions?

She scrunched her eyebrows together. "No, Dakota isn't so upset about it, not to *that* degree," she said. "I just told her we go to heaven when we die, and she was fine."

I would ask a couple more parents and get similar answers. There were no simple answers for Finn, though. There never have been.

At the kitchen table, Finn munched on French fries, then looked up at me. "I never want to have any kids," she said between bites.

"Really? Why is that?"

"I would be too afraid one would kill the other."

I dropped my sandwich on the plate, appetite a distant memory now. "That would never happen, and you will not kill anyone, either."

I watched her eyes become glassy with tears. "You don't know that for sure."

"Yes, I do," I insisted.

"How? How do you know it?"

Around in a circle we went. I assured while she dug the OCD hole deeper. I would later come to understand that all my assurances meant that I had a shovel as well and although I didn't know it at the time, I was right beside her making that pit even harder to climb out of. I was enabling.

"Promise me I'm not a bad person."

"I swear you aren't."

My fear of sending her to a therapist was also tempered by the knowledge that the Harm OCD I had experienced as a teenager had gone away on its own after a few tormenting months. I hoped that Finn's would do the same.

She eventually stopped talking about it. I was afraid to ask if it had gone away for fear that if it had, my asking about it would reawaken it. However, more compulsions emerged. For example, excessive hand-washing took hold. Her hands felt like sandpaper, and then they began to crack and bleed.

"Have you seen her hands?" I asked Sean one evening as Finn paced her bedroom floor.

"Yeah, she's washing them too much."

"It's clearly OCD."

"Everybody's so obsessed with germs."

"Well, I think they talk about it at school so much that it kind of pushes the obsessive kids over the microbial edge. She just seems so stressed out."

"Yeah, but nobody's beating her or screaming at her."

As a combat veteran, his idea of stress differed greatly from that of an adolescent girl with OCD. He had never suffered with such compulsions, either. It wasn't his fault that he couldn't understand. I felt I needed to push harder. "It's like she doesn't enjoy anything anymore. It makes me sad. Do you remember when she used to join all kinds of teams and made friends so easy?"

He smiled. "Yeah, within a few minutes of being at the playground, she would make a friend." My mind went back to happier days when she would hang from the monkey bars talking to a new friend. She had no problem asking other kids to play. They would chase and laugh. I remembered sunny days and picnics in the park. How did I go from that to having a fifth grader that experienced a level of stress that people four times her age might not even experience? OCD is a thief.

"I guess all kids get moody and lose that happy-go-lucky joy of childhood at some point. But she comes home crying so often and worries herself sick about whether she's offended one of her friends or said the wrong thing." Making sure I had his attention, I said, "I think she might need to talk to someone. Maybe we're just too close to the situation. You know how kids are. Sometimes somebody else can say the same thing to them and they respond better because it isn't coming from their parents. Maybe she would get something out of talking to a therapist."

Sean thought about that for a moment before responding. "Well, I guess you could go online and see who takes our insurance."

I searched through one database after another, hoping to find a specialist in OCD. The research I had done stated that it was important to find someone with experience and expertise treating OCD specifically. I learned later that the list of things a therapist says they treat isn't necessarily their area of expertise, nor does it mean they've ever treated anyone with that disorder. It just means they are familiar with it. I was convinced Finn had OCD, but most of the psychologists and therapists who specialized in it were out of network, too far away, or completely booked up.

Also, many didn't take insurance, but would instead have you pay out of pocket and then would provide us with a "super bill" to submit to our insurance in hopes that they would cover a portion of it. I understand this. The practitioners are trying their best to see as many patients as possible while dealing with endless billing as well. After speaking with a friend who handles billing for a therapist, I see that they truly want to help and struggle with insurance as well. It's tough all the way around. I don't know the answer.

I've asked myself more than once what in the world parents did for their children suffering with OCD, or any mental illness, if they couldn't pay out of pocket. If it was this hard for someone with coverage and a little money in a health savings account to find help, what did the rest of these parents do? What did this mean for people who direly needed help?

I had mentioned the idea of a therapist to Finn more and more over the past few months. At first, she really felt nervous about telling a stranger such personal things. I even suggested that she didn't have to tell them things that she was uncomfortable with. In hindsight, perhaps I should have pushed her a little more, but I wanted to get her in the door to begin with. To be fair, there was also a part of me that still feared her telling the therapist about the Harm OCD. At any rate, her hands weren't getting any better. She hated when I put lotion on them, so I would often wait until she fell asleep and then coat them with ointment. Thank God she was a heavy sleeper.

There were no psychologists immediately available; their waiting lists were long. We ended up choosing a therapist who had a degree as a licensed social worker. I discovered she was one of the few who had availability in our area.

The day of her first appointment, I glanced at Finn in the passenger's seat as we drove to the office. "How're you doing over there?"

"A little nervous."

"I think it will be helpful, though."

"Yeah, I think so, too."

"Just remember, there's not much you could say that would shock her. She's been counseling for years. I'm sure she's heard it all by this point."

"Yeah."

I still didn't want to tell her outright that she should mention the thoughts of harming someone. Even though I knew I'd had it, gotten past it, and never hurt a soul, I had never heard the term Harm OCD at that point. However, I knew that many people with OCD suffered from intrusive thoughts, and I assumed the scary thoughts of harming someone was part of that.

We walked into the building to find a calming atmosphere with soft music playing and comfortable surroundings. When Leah came out to meet us, she had a kind smile and a soothing voice. She walked us back to her office, where she explained that whatever was said between her and Finn would stay between them unless there was specific talk of committing suicide or harming herself. Finn was still a minor at that point, and while Leah didn't want to betray her trust, I understood that she still had a legal obligation to warn me and Sean if there was an imminent threat.

Leah explained, "There's a distinction between saying you've thought of suicide and you're *planning* on killing yourself. Everyone has thought of something like that, at least fleetingly. That doesn't mean they want to do it. Does that make sense to everyone?"

"Of course," I replied while looking at Finn and hoping that this distinction would also translate to Finn's understanding of thoughts being different than intentions when it came to the scary images popping into her head. After this introduction, I went back out to the waiting room and left Finn and Leah to talk on their own.

After the session, Finn shared some with me about what they discussed. The therapist felt the handwashing wasn't about cleanliness but a subconscious desire to keep her anxiety from infecting other people. Finn never told this therapist about the Harm OCD. Believing her condition was no more serious than a little excessive handwashing, the therapist assured Finn that she just had too much stress and anxiety. They met for three months with no effect.

Finn would have massive breakdowns in front of me, often sobbing inconsolably on the floor for an hour or longer, telling me she was depressed and found no joy in life. She would tell me she was afraid she was a worthless person, but she wouldn't bring up the source of her meltdowns to Leah. When I'd asked Finn about what Leah said concerning these episodes, she would tell me that, during her therapy sessions, she would forget to mention them. Finally, after three months, Leah ended the weekly appointments, telling Finn, "Just call me if you need anything else."

She spent months in therapy with no improvement. I remember the night Finn told me that Leah didn't think it was OCD, but stress.

"I disagree. If you panic when you try to stop washing your hands and only washing them relieves the panic, then it's more than stress. Intrusive thoughts are part of OCD as well. Perhaps if you'd mention that to her . . ."

"Mom, they talked about OCD at health class in school. Those people have to have everything neat, and I'm not like that. I'm not neat. I'm certainly not organized."

"Oh, I know. We've met." I laughed. "I've seen your room. But OCD isn't about neatness. That's a total misunderstanding. It's about an overwhelming compulsion to do something and not being able to stop without feeling panicked or believing something horrible will happen unless you do things a certain way. Like washing your hands or when you have scary thoughts and having to replace it with a good thought or touch a certain object while thinking a good thought to banish the scary thought or whatever. I don't have to tell you. You know all about it. The neatness is a cliché."

Therein lies the danger of the "neatness" misunderstanding about OCD, though someone could have a compulsion associated with neatness, we have to stop using this as some sort of criteria. She believed she didn't have it and no longer needed therapy because she was misled at school by a teacher about what OCD was. This is dangerous.

I could tell we were just getting irritated with each other, so I let it go. For a couple of years, Finn didn't mention the Harm OCD to me, and right or wrong, I didn't ask. I was far too scared of activating it if it had gone dormant, as mine had when I was younger, or making it worse.

## Finn says:

A while after the first incident, my Harm OCD calmed down on its own, probably because it eventually faded from my mind, and other things distracted me. I wish I could say that I was free from it for a few years, but that could not be further from the truth. It simply took other forms, some big ones being hand-washing, morality, and following orders.

First was the handwashing. To be perfectly honest, I am not a very neat or even a clean person. My room is always a mess, my binder is never organized, and I always forget to throw away the trash in my room. But after my sister was born, my parents emphasized washing my hands often so I wouldn't get her sick, which makes sense and is reasonable, but my OCD took that and applied it to everything, and soon I was washing my hands all the time because I did not want to get other people sick. This doesn't sound bad, but my definition of what was clean and was not differed greatly from other people's.

For example, when you go to the bathroom, you pull your pants up before you wash your hands, but in my brain that means the waistband of my pants is always contaminated, and the bottom of my shirt touches my pants so that is dirty, too. My shirt moves around and makes the entire rim of my jeans polluted, including my pockets, so now I can't touch any of these things without feeling as though my hands are horribly dirty, and I am going to get someone sick because they don't know how disgusting I am. I still struggle with handwashing to this day. My hands are constantly dried out, and on the worst occasions they crack and bleed.

Morality is a bit more self-explanatory; I could do nothing that might be bad, no breaking rules, no matter how big or small. I always had to do what was considered polite or thoughtful, even if I did not want to. A large part of my identity rested on how nice and considerate I was because that was what they always praised me for, so I constantly had to act that way or else there was something wrong with me.

If I accidentally did something off, for example, if I said something that could be slightly rude or taken the wrong way, I would have to explain, apologize a million times, then kick myself so I didn't make that error again. It did not help that, thanks to Catholic school, I had the threat of eternal damnation over my head if I made a mistake. But here is a quick fact about OCD and strict religions: they don't mix, or, depending on your viewpoint, they mix too well, much to my displeasure. I don't think my Catholic upbringing did me any favors.

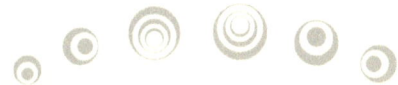

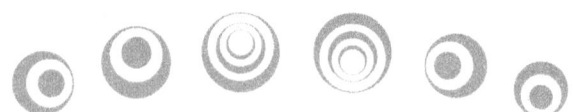

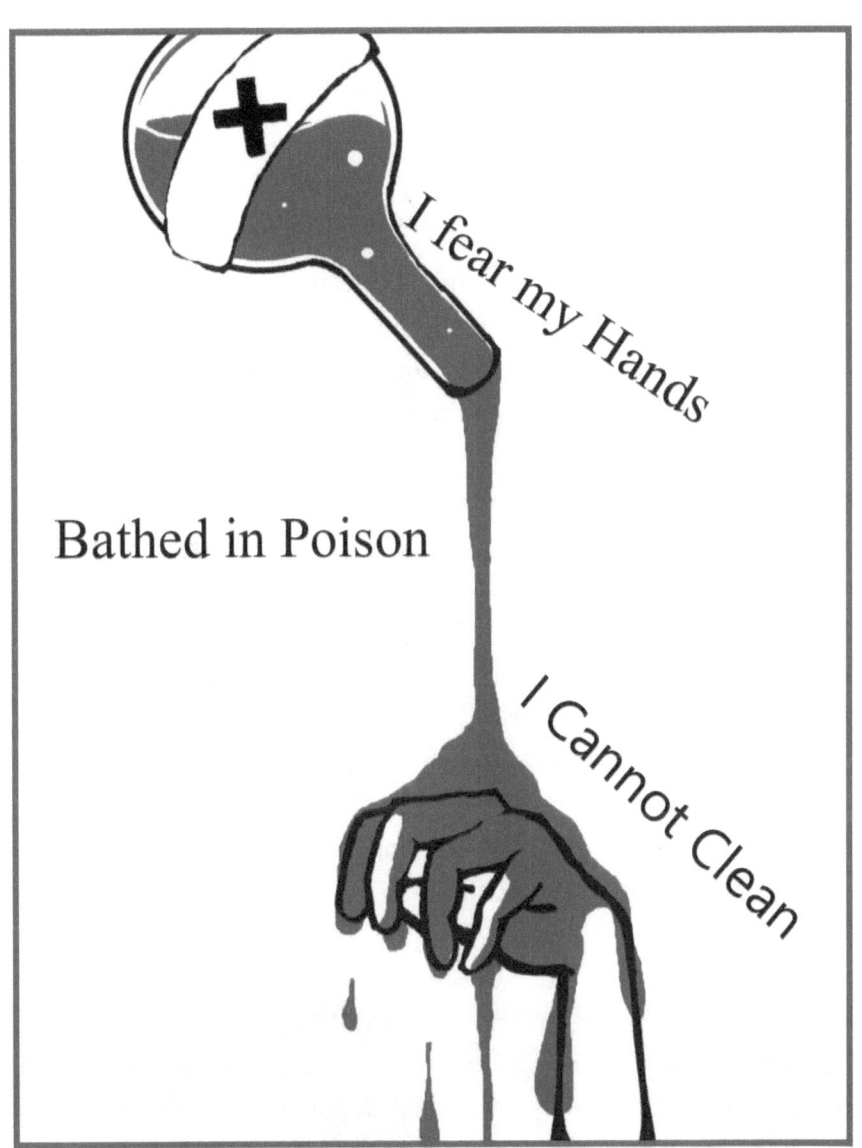

I fear my Hands

Bathed in Poison

I Cannot Clean

**Illustration by Finn Conrey**

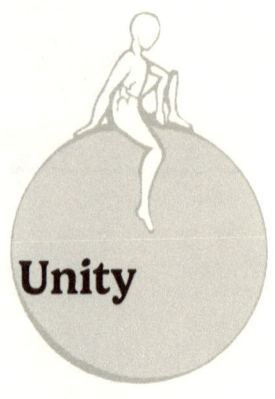

## Unity

# CHAPTER 5

When Brea was six months old and Finn was eleven, we moved from our small ranch house to a larger home just a couple of miles away. It was a beautiful neighborhood with lots of trees and a little pond. Finn had participated in the neighborhood's swim team for several years, so by the time we bought a house there, it already felt like home. With a little more room to spread out, we were no longer bumping into each other in the kitchen. However, a move is a stressful thing, especially for someone with OCD. While sitting in our home office, Sean and I heard thumps coming from the ceiling. They went from one side to the other and back again. When Finn came down for dinner later, Sean and I asked her what was going on.

"Oh, I didn't know you heard that. The pacing soothes my nerves."

"Well, I've heard Michael J. Fox paces," I said, and then explained who he was to my daughter. "Many people believe pacing stirs up creativity." I was trying to skew positive.

The carpet quickly became matted and flattened by relentless worry, making its way out of her body and onto the floor where it became crushed by her burden. We eventually got used to the pacing. It became background noise, like the hum of a refrigerator. She paced in the morning, after lunch, before bed, and to decompress after a trip outside the house.

By this point she was in middle school and the kids were judgier. I remembered my own middle school experience. I'd always felt that it was far worse than elementary or high school. The kids were just old enough to know that they had the power to alienate and bully those that were different but not mature enough to understand how mean and obnoxious they were being. Between Finn's undiagnosed OCD and her suspicion that she felt different from the other kids without knowing exactly why, she became more and more isolated. The friendships she'd experienced as a child fell by the wayside. She eventually became so miserable that we enrolled her a hybrid Christian homeschool in hopes that not having the pressure of heading into school to deal with intense social situations every day would be a better setup for someone dealing with so much stress and anxiety. She went to school two days a week and worked from home the other three.

But even at the new school, the problems seemed to follow her. There was difficulty relating to the other kids and the sense that she didn't quite fit in. There were some friendly students there, but she didn't make any close friends despite joining various groups.

### Finn says:

When I was in 8th grade, I was in a Christian school, and every day the whole school would gather for morning prayer. One day, while we were finishing our prayer, I had an invasive thought and instead of praying to God, I accidentally prayed to Slenderman. (Slenderman was a popular monster and horror game character from the late 2000s.) I had just prayed to a fictional murderer! Even though he was fictional, the murder part made me feel horrified and disgusted with myself. I was worried I was going to hell. It was an accident, but that didn't matter to me. My fate was almost sealed.

I thought, maybe, just maybe, if I prayed for forgiveness, explained myself, and promised to try to never do it again, I would be forgiven. There was just one problem. For some reason, I thought if there are spiritual energies in the world and auras and such, maybe that energy could bind itself to the exact molecules that surround me and those that I was touching as the terrible prayer happened. These molecules would remember the sin I committed and hold a record of it. This meant I would need to stand in the same spot as before to undo what I did, in the exact position, and I could not move until I had fixed it. I know that sounds odd, but I thought it was better to be safe than spend the rest of eternity in hell with God hating me. I also know it seems weird that a Christian would think about spiritual energies and auras, but my family was already pretty progressive, as far as Christians go.

So, once I finished the first prayer, I tried to go back and re-pray to undo my mistake. But because I had to stand in the exact same spot, I got a lot of weird looks from teachers and classmates. I was so embarrassed, but I couldn't explain myself. There was also a strict time limit because class was about to start. I was so stressed and panicked, but I had to do it, and the longer I stood there, the weirder it got for onlookers. If you know anything about invasive thoughts, you also know the more you think about them, the more they keep popping up. The more I tried to fix it, the more I screwed it up! Eventually, after yet another invasive thought, I prayed quickly, apologizing for my thoughts, and I ran off before I could think any more bad ones.

After that, I began to worry about the next time I prayed, and the time after that, and the time after that. Praying became a fearful event for me. I worried I would accidentally pray to someone I didn't want to, doom myself, and disappoint God. This continued for at least half a year. Eventually I would settle into a routine of "Hi, God, love you. Please protect my family. Gotta go before I accidentally do something bad. Thank you!" But throughout the whole prayer, I would get little blips of intrusive thoughts and try my best to speed past them, and if too much of the badness got through before I could continue praying, I would have to start over. It was a very stressful ordeal. I always worried I was somehow demonic or doomed or unworthy of God's love or an awful person. I am grateful to know in retrospect that it is not that way at all.

But sadly, part of the ritual carried on into the future. When I would have a bad intrusive thought, I would have to stay in the same spot or touch the same thing while thinking a good thought and making it clear that the other thought I had was not reflective of who I was as a person.

Sometimes I could find a little peace when I got lost in a drawing.

Art became a refuge for Finn. She discovered she had a genuine talent for sketching. I looked on in wonder at the drawings coming from her amazing imagination, characters that materialized from inside her mind. She had a knack for animation. Whether it was purposeful or not, she gravitated toward the different and strangely beautiful. I loved and admired that about her.

A couple of years passed with Finn having tearful meltdowns on a loop. I felt helpless and desperate for solutions. The counseling had done little good, and she went back and forth about the prospect of seeing another professional. I waited and hoped and held onto the idea that as her brain developed things would get better.

Sean was working a lot of overtime, and I was logging many hours per week dashing from one side of town to the other. I dropped Finn off at school, then Brea at her pre-K program. During that window, I would try to get caught up on chores and, if I had time, even go for a run. Three hours later, I picked Brea up from school, and we rushed to make her speech therapy appointment across town. As soon as we finished there, it was time to pick up Finn.

She eventually became miserable at her new hybrid school. The teachers and staff were very conservative, and it bothered her that they openly condemned homosexuality. I believe she knew, if only on a subconscious level, that she was queer, but, queer or straight, Finn was always one to fight for someone's right to be different. She's courageous in that way, courage that takes many people a lifetime to build. But at fourteen, school is all about fitting in, and Finn was born to stand out. At 5'10" she stood out anyway, but her personality did as well.

She joined JROTC while at the hybrid school. I couldn't help but notice she gravitated toward anything that helped her relate to her father. He was a veteran of both the Marine Corps and Army, and she was very proud of him. When she was little, she would shovel her meals into her mouth so quickly I feared she would choke. When I asked her about this later, she told me that she'd noticed how fast her dad ate—a leftover from his Marine Corps days of having to eat quickly during boot camp as you never knew when the drill sergeant was going to walk in and end mealtime without warning, thus the best strategy was to eat fast.

There were a few good days of JROTC. I'd pull up on a crisp fall day and see them in formation, or fresh from a workout and she seemed happy to be there, at least on some level, but soon enough, she saw injustices that stressed her out. There was a kid who didn't keep up well with the physical rigors of the group or the teasing forays stemming from the toxic masculinity that many of the cadets engaged in. Finn went to the commander, a retired Air Force colonel, and told him the young man was being harassed. The commander confronted the boy that had done the hazing, but when the adults had their backs turned, the cadet in charge gave them all a speech about snitches. Finn didn't stay, and I couldn't blame her. It was too bad; they could have used a cadet like her, but she would never be one to just fall in line and ignore injustice, and I didn't expect her to.

Though JROTC didn't turn out to be who she was, identifying someone in need and courageously defending him, even knowing it might cost her friends or standing among the cadets, defined and shaped exactly who Finn was more than the program itself ever could have. She didn't need to stay with it forever, only long enough to find out who she was, and she did. Success isn't always measured in finishing but what you do while you're there.

Being totally disillusioned with the conservative school that promoted traditional roles for girls (though they were allowed to join JROTC) was depressing for Finn. She discussed the idea of attending public high school. With the immaturity of middle school students no longer a factor and Finn slowly realizing who she was, public school became a better option. We live in a fairly diverse area, and the high school in our district is by far the most diverse. Finn was excited to meet students of all kinds.

Almost immediately, she began to gravitate toward the kids who were transgender, gay, or bisexual, even though she had not yet come out to them or me. In these groups, she found kindred spirits. And it would oversimplify the situation, and the kids, to say that it was only because she was discovering she was queer. Finn found mutual admiration in this group of people who weren't afraid to embrace who they were, or if they were afraid, they were embracing it anyway. Brave is more valuable than fearless. It's harder won.

Though it was difficult for her to maintain friendships with OCD, making her question every move she made, one friendship during that time endured. Her friend Vincent became a constant in her life. The three of us even attended the 2019 Atlanta Pride Run in Piedmont Park together. There were all kinds of people there, so diverse and beautiful. It was such a joy to see a group of individuals being exactly who they were and being accepted for it. Everyone there was so supportive and kind. I know she won't find that type of atmosphere all the time or everywhere she goes, but I pray she finds it when she needs it.

Not long after Finn changed schools, she and I sat on the couch enjoying the quiet. The TV was off, and the Christmas tree was twinkling. Brea was already in bed, and I was beginning to wind down when I noticed Finn was shaking.

"What's wrong, sweetie? Are you feeling okay?"

"There's something I have to tell you."

I was fairly certain I knew what it was, and I wanted to rush in and say it for her, but I didn't. I knew there would be other times when she'd have to say it when she knew, before the words were uttered, that she would be rejected, made fun of, or told she was going to hell. I wouldn't be doing her any favors to charge in and rescue her now. I owed her the gift of knowing she could speak her truth here, where she would be accepted. She could say it here to someone who's spent her whole life telling her that it's a bravery for a person to live their truth, not a curse, not a disease, and certainly not a sin. Still, I felt like a caged lioness that couldn't reach her cub when it needed her. The silence stretched out impossibly long, though it was only seconds.

Finally, I heard what I expected. "Mom, I think I'm bisexual or gay."

I told her how proud I was to be her mom. She leaned her head on my shoulder, and we talked well into the night.

### Finn says:

When I was younger, I never thought I was gay, but when I was in middle school I began to wonder if I was. I quickly came to the "conclusion" I was overreacting. In all actuality, I came to no definitive conclusion and was tired of trying to figure it out. I had other bouts of questioning and things I should have taken as signs, like the time my mom asked me what type of boys I liked, and I could think of no traits in particular, so I just said, "dark hair" and left it at that.

I finally started to seriously question it in 11th grade. At the time, I wasn't even aware of why I questioned it. I just did. You may wonder why I didn't reach this point sooner? A large reason was because the middle school I was in was very homophobic. For example, a girl I went to school with stopped watching *Doctor Who* because one of the Doctor's companions was gay. Another reason I didn't arrive at this question earlier was because anytime I started having natural intimate fantasies, I would have a wave of religious fear triggered by my OCD, and I would have to pray, say it was a moment of weakness, and then promise God to try not to do it again.

When I actually started down this path of true self-awareness, it was fairly slow going for a few months, I would just think about it for a while and then I would say to myself. *Well, that was interesting, but you can't actually be gay because you are straight. Yep, the fact that you have never had a real crush on a guy that you did not make yourself think about in order to fit in means nothing. Definitely no repressed emotions here!* Then I would shove all of that back in the closet. I definitely think besides compulsory heterosexuality, there was also an OCD component to it. After every debate with myself, I had to mentally assure myself that I was straight, and if I said or thought about it too much, then something bad would happen. Did I even know what that was? Absolutely not. Did it matter? No, I was questioning everything, and that was scary. But slowly I started to open to the idea more and more.

After a while of this. I finally did something that scared me to try to figure it out. I was sitting on the bus heading home from school, and I told myself, *All right, I'm gonna sit here for a few seconds and think, Okay I am straight for the rest of my life, how does that feel? And then I am gonna sit here for a few seconds and think, Okay I am gay for the rest of my life, how does that feel?* So, I sat through the straight part, and didn't feel much because I was worrying about what the gay part was gonna feel like. So, I sat there for a second and then began going through the thought exercise, "Okay, I am gay . . . HOLY SHIT! I'M GAY!" The realization hit me all at once, the label felt right and everything began to fit, and it was not an intrusive thought like my regular thoughts but an actual realization. Then I began worrying, *Wait! Wait! Wait! This is all a misunderstanding, there is no way I can be gay! I am just overreacting. This is just an exercise.* But at that point I couldn't shove it all back in the box (or the closet, if you will) so I just had to wait till the bus reached my stop, and then I had to go home and figure out what to do with myself. I tried to deny it a little longer. Eventually, I got hit with the non-intrusive thought of one of my female classmates being really cute, and I hoped she thought I was cute, too. By then, I just accepted that I was gay or at the very least a 95/5 bisexual kinda mix, given a very specific kind of guy (we can at least call me queer as a catch all) because I realized that there was no going back because I had never been straight to begin with.

When Finn came out, I couldn't wait for her to get involved in groups that would help her navigate her newfound identity. She was no longer comfortable at the Catholic church and had railed against having to attend confirmation classes. She believed that the confirmation obligation was a way to "hold our faith hostage from us." As frustrating as it was to have to beg her to finish, I couldn't help but smile to myself. I love a good rebel. Jesus was a rebel, despite the white washing that has been applied through the ages. He was walking around, ticking people off in his day, challenging the status quo. So does Finn. Though she finished her Catholic classes, after confirmation, she refused to return.

"Those people make me feel bad. They tell me that God is loving but then say you have to follow all these rules to please God. Their rules."

"I understand, but I take what works for me and leave the rest," I told her. "Those priests and teachers are still people with opinions, prejudices, and faults just like anyone else. Your spirituality is between you and God."

"Then why am I supposed to confess to a priest?"

"You don't have to. You can just talk to God."

She began sobbing. "But they make me feel bad if I don't."

"You shouldn't feel bad. Catholicism is not for everyone. Just talk to God. He's not mad at you. You kick ass and he knows it. Just like I know it. You're awesome."

I realized the OCD and religion were getting all tangled up again. Religion can be a tough pill to swallow even without OCD, but with it, it can be a nightmare of fear and moral scrupulosity. Not only that, but it was also easier for me to take what worked and leave the rest because I wasn't walking into a church building knowing that a majority of the congregation, usually including the pastor or priest, already held something against me. I wasn't queer. Try as I may, I would never be able to entirely understand it from her experience.

"Well, listen, I've been wanting to try that Unitarian church not far from here. Why don't we go check that out?"

She agreed, and we went for a Sunday morning service. One of the first things the pastor said was, "You aren't broken. You aren't stained or wretched. This life is God doing business in the world as you."

As he spoke, my mind drifted back to a night in a friend's driveway watching the sky for shooting stars through their telescope. His sweet little boys took turns looking through the telescope then turned to look at their dad, and one of them said, "If we look through this telescope, will we be able to see God?"

He smiled. "All you need to do to see God is look at each other."

They both giggled and went on about their business. Perhaps it was lost on them at the moment, but it wasn't lost on me. I firmly believe it.

Everything the Unitarian pastor said was a breath of fresh air, and, honestly, he was simply telling me things that I already felt from going to churches, taking what worked and leaving the rest, as was my heathen way, and combining it with what I already knew to be true. In the quiet, still moments, when everything was broken, burned away, there existed one simple truth: love trumps dogma. Whether it's a rebellious streak or just some wiring in my head that isn't as scared of damnation as one should be, I've never been afraid to embrace what God means to *me* and let the rest go.

But what impressed me the most was the day that two women who had married each other walked up front with the LGBTQ rainbow flag and invited the congregation to their meeting that they held once a month for the "LGBTQ and Friends" luncheon. I knew that this was the kind of open-minded and welcoming place where Finn and I could be at peace attending. Not only that, but I was also surprised that one of the women that spoke was a member of the writer's critique group that I attended. She wrote wonderful Southern short stories. Her presence was a piece of synchronicity that made me feel like I was on the right track.

A couple of months later, Finn attended the luncheon with me. They couldn't have been more welcoming and tolerant of me having to bring Brea, now six, to the meeting with us as Sean was working. They recommended that we attend the local Parents and Friends of Lesbians and Gays (PFLAG) meeting as there weren't any young people in the LGBTQ organization at the church.

PFLAG was wonderful. It was uplifting to be around other parents and a few kids as well, who could talk about the issues and challenges that went along with coming out or supporting a friend or family member as they do so.

Not long after attending the meeting, Finn and I got a call from Drea, a member of LGBTQ and Friends. After a few pleasantries she explained, "I recently attended a Coming Out Monologues at a library. Parents, children, family and various other members of the community got up and spoke about their experience of coming out or what it was like for their children to come out. I was really touched by the honesty and awareness there. I was thinking it would be a wonderful experience for our spiritual community. Would you and Finn be willing to attend and share a brief monologue from your perspectives?"

"I'd love to. This is a great idea!"

"Excellent! I thought of you and Finn when I heard about this. I think it would be wonderful to have parent and child pairs speak. Do you think Finn would be willing to participate as well?"

"I'm sure she would, but I'll ask her."

I hung up the phone and told Finn all about it. She seemed enthused, and I was excited by the idea that other people from the LGBTQ community would be there, likely many younger people as well. I really wanted her to meet people she could relate to.

Finn and I had both written monologues to read, but as the day neared, Finn got increasingly frightened of having to read in front of the group.

"But, Finn, you said you wanted to meet more people like you and make more friends. This will be the perfect opportunity. These folks are more on your side than just about any place."

"I know. I know. It just . . . I don't know. It makes me panic. But I'm afraid you are going to be disappointed in me if I don't go."

"I won't be disappointed in you. It just seems like it could be helpful."

I didn't say any more about it. You can only encourage a person so much before they begin to feel that they are being pushed, and when they feel pushed, they tend to push back.

She attended the short "dress rehearsal." They were doing the monologues black box theater style with a solid dark backdrop, a single spotlight in a dark room, and a stool where the speaker sits. They wanted to work with the lighting while people practiced reading their monologues. Finn was very withdrawn and barely spoke when the other speakers attempted to talk to her. Again, I felt like I was walking the line between pushing just enough, but not so much that it backfired. I desperately wanted her to have more fellowship with kindred spirits.

The night of the monologues came, and I stood in the living room with my purse on my shoulder reminding myself not to push too much. "Are you sure you don't want to go?"

"Yeah, I'm sure. I just don't want you to be disappointed in me."

"I'm not. I promise. You know where your limits are." I tried to sound upbeat. There was no sense in making her feel bad. "Thanks for watching your sister."

"Sure. Have fun."

I drove to the church feeling sad. When I arrived, there was a bigger crowd than I expected. Drea, the organizer from LGBTQ and friends, was the first to say hello. She has a kind soul and soothing presence.

"I'm sorry but Finn can't make it tonight. She just got too nervous. I told her she didn't even have to read, but . . ."

"Oh no. I wish I'd have known. I could have talked with her."

"Thank you. I'm not sure it would have helped. She was just too anxiety ridden about it."

"Okay. Maybe next time. We want to do this again. Please tell her I missed her. You know, you were the first person I called. I wasn't sure this idea was going to work, and when you were so enthused about it, it made me believe others might be, too."

"Are you kidding? This is an awesome idea!"

She spotted more people she needed to chat with, and I was happy to see a few of my friends were there as well: my dear friend Kathy, her husband Ed, and George from our critique group. Having their support was everything, not only because I had to read about something so personal in front of everyone but also because I carried deep sorrow in my chest about Finn not being present.

My heart pounded as I read the monologue I'd written, expressing the thoughts of being the mother of a child who'd recently come out. But even as I read, I mourned the fact that Finn wasn't there with me.

The audience was kind and attentive as I read:

*"I remember when my daughter told me, 'Mom, I'm gay.' I told her how courageous she was, and how proud I was to be her mom.*

*"There have been so many brave LGBTQ souls who came before us, when it wasn't so safe to live one's truth. When I consider the Stone Wall uprising and the marches that followed and those who've lost jobs, reputations, and even lost their lives to make it possible for me to raise my queer daughter in more safety, acceptance, and love, I'm grateful. And this wonderful fellowship here at Unity provides a place where no one is going to tell my daughter she's in rebellion to the will of God, that she's going to hell, that there's something wrong with her. I know she can live her spirituality here with total acceptance. I don't want my daughter to be simply tolerated. I want her to be accepted and celebrated as she truly is. This place is a sharp contrast to the churches I grew up in,*

*where being gay was considered a sin, something to scream about from the pulpit. I may one day march back into one of those churches and say, 'Here I am, and I've brought my big queer daughter with me. Deal with it.' I have such gratitude in my heart for this beautiful, welcoming, inclusive atmosphere here. Thank you."*

I went back to my seat and settled in to hear the rest of the speakers take their place in the spotlight and tell their stories.

There were tales that broke my heart: parents who disowned their children, brothers and sisters who no longer spoke, and even the story of a brother who wished he could return the kidney his lesbian sister had so compassionately given him years earlier. One by one they revealed their beautiful—and sometimes, broken—spirits.

There were even members of the LGBTQ club from Kennesaw State University where Finn attended as a dual enrollment student for her senior year of high school, telling stories and taking part in the question-and-answer period. I'd been telling her she should check out their club for a while. Participating in the monologues would have been a way to meet some members before going to the group. But her OCD mixing itself in with a heaping dose of social anxiety—one fueling the other—had kept Finn from the very thing that could have helped her.

As I drove home, considering all the persecution the older LGBTQ folks in the group had gone through, I shuddered at what would have happened to my compassionate, beautiful daughter if she'd been born decades earlier. If having OCD didn't get her completely shunned from society, being queer would have.

I pulled into the driveway and thanked God for progress and compassion. What could I tell Finn about the meeting without making her feel bad about not attending? Frustration rose in my chest as I grieved her missing the evening. Did I handle this right? Yet I knew showing this frustration would only alienate her more. Someone who's already suffering shouldn't be made to feel guilty as well.

I took a deep breath and got out of my car to head up the stairs. I heard Finn and Brea on the floor above me, watching TV.

"Hi, sweeties. Did you two have a good evening?"

"Yup, just watching TV. How did it go?"

"Great! There were even some people there representing the LGBTQ group at KSU. They had a panel answer questions from the audience after everyone read their monologues. I think I have a better understanding of what nonbinary is now. A KSU student explained it to an audience member who asked. There were some really awesome people there. Tomorrow I'll have to tell you some more of the stories I heard."

"I hope you aren't upset at me for not going."

"No, I understand. Everyone is at a different place. I get it."

"Okie dokie," she said and went back to looking at her phone as I told Brea it was time for bed.

Finn said no more about it that evening. The next day we talked about all the great, and often sorrowful, stories I'd heard that night. But I said no more about her not going; it would only have made her feel bad. We had gone through it already. I still couldn't help but think, though, that I wish she'd gone. Maybe I should have told her to just attend and never pushed the idea of her reading the monologue. Maybe I pushed her too much. What is too much?

Of all the things I was grateful for that night, all the brave souls who got up to speak, the inclusive, accepting atmosphere, from the audience as well as those brave enough to answer questions and educate people, I never applied that gentle gratitude to myself. *Progress and compassion* applied to me too, but it was harder to see for myself.

Sometimes we only notice in hindsight that we're doing the best we can.

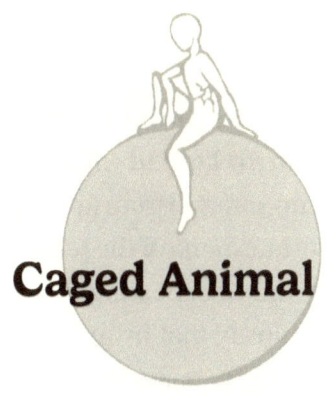

# CHAPTER 6

# Caged Animal

During Finn's senior year while attending Kennesaw State University as a dual enrollment student, she would sometimes be wildly anxiety-ridden or in tears when I picked her up from school. Concentrating became difficult when the OCD thoughts arose. She sometimes got stuck in a loop when reading a certain passage and had to go back and read it again, or the certainty that something was very, very bad would happen plagued her until she gave in.

It's amazing that not only can OCD be handed down genetically, but the kinds of OCD family members experience seem to be handed down as well. I'd had similar thoughts when reading a book. I would zone out for a couple of sentences, as anyone does now and then while reading. However, I would get the sudden notion that if I didn't go back and read the passage again while paying perfect attention, it meant that I would get cancer. For a while, it made reading a book difficult. So much for reading to relax. The frustration became so great that I eventually refused to go back and read the passages again several times. I breathed deeply and talked myself out of reading it again. Yet, my eyes started drifting back up the page to try to read it. *But you'll get cancer if you don't.* Eventually, I got better at not "obeying" the OCD. There was a lot of panicking involved: sweating palms, pounding heart, and fear.

I would later come to realize I was intuitively conducting my own Cognitive Behavioral Therapy (CBT). More specifically, it was the use of Exposure and Response Prevention (ERP) therapy. Although I had never heard of ERP at the time, it just made sense to me to train myself *not* to do it. But to be clear, I do not believe that everyone can or should conduct their own ERP therapy without a professional. I was just at a point in my life and with my OCD where I could handle it.

Finn suffered from intense morality OCD as well. She would ask too many questions of the teacher to make sure she was doing something right and not cheating *in any way* by omission or lack of clarity. The scrupulosity that brings the sufferer to tears can make those around them angry, believing that the questioner is being purposely difficult and holding up the class. It could be anything from being afraid of using the wrong source for a project or hearing a due date but still having this nagging sense in the back of her brain that she didn't hear it right, and now the teacher is going to be angry or something horrific will happen if she doesn't include or exclude the right thing.

### Finn says:

When it comes to following orders, I had to do everything just right so I was as good, helpful, and nice as I could be, which ties back into my Morality OCD. So, when people gave me directions, I clarified them over and over just to make sure that I was doing everything right, and I spent all of my energy trying to make sure it was perfect. I would even come back to stuff later that I was worried I didn't do just right. This process annoyed me and the person that had given me the orders. But when I got things done right, it reinforced the OCD, and it made people trust me more, so they gave me more to do, which continued the vicious cycle.

I was driving back and forth to take Finn to her classes at KSU as she only had her learner's permit and was now a full-time college student. Brea was now seven years old and in elementary school. We had to time out Finn's classes so that I could get back and forth across town after carpool at the elementary school. Brea's speech was finally coming along well, but she still had issues explaining what she did during the school day. Therefore, I was hesitant to let her ride the school bus, knowing that if an incident occurred, it would be difficult for her to tell me what had happened.

Brea sat in the back seat playing on my phone as Finn got in the car and slammed the door. A storm cloud of heavy OCD energy was looking to burst forth at the slightest touch or sound. I wanted to ask. I didn't want to ask. At some point we all have to deal with crisis on our own. But I'm her mother, and I always want to help, to protect, to fix. Knowing when to intervene is a conundrum for any mother, but for the mother with a child plagued by OCD, it blurs the lines even further.

Finally, I said, "What's wrong, sweetie?"

"I don't know. Well . . ." She struggled to put the book-laden backpack at her feet, but her long legs filled the space. She shoved it past her legs and to the floor with a growl. I knew my signal to keep quiet. A minute went by before she spoke.

"This girl that I had been partnered with before for projects asked me something, but I was embarrassed because I couldn't tell what she said, then when I worked up the courage to ask her what she said, it would have been weird to ask because too much time had passed by. Now she thinks I purposely ignored her. She thinks I don't like her. I don't know how to make friends anymore. How do you, like, *do* that?"

"You just talk. It tends to come about organically."

"Well, I don't know what to say, and she thinks I'm a jerk now."

"I think it is in your nature to make friends and be friendly. You were never a shy child. Your anxiety is just making everything seem harder than it is."

"Yeah."

I never wanted "yeah" to be the end of anything. I wanted to keep talking until she felt better, but conversations stemming from anxiety and OCD tend to go in a circle. Sometimes they even spool up the anxiety. I'll tell her how much I believe in her or how I know she can do something, and she will get more frustrated and tell me I don't understand, when I've been through these things myself. I imagine most parents can relate to this scenario: metal health issues or not.

## Finn says:

Though I was dealing with major anxiety in college, there were some supportive students there and earlier in high school. They understand mental illness and have an openness about it that the older generation simply does not have.

Often, when you go talk to an older person, mainly boomers or gen x, about mental health, there is a weird amount of unease, wariness and occasionally fear. Even though mental health has become more common to talk about, it is hard to erase years of having it stigmatized and mocked openly in casual conversation. In fact, a lot of these people are trying to be better and more open, but they cannot talk about it casually just yet, sometimes even when they or a loved one are afflicted. They dance around the topic like it is something to be feared or something that can only be treated with seriousness. While I do believe that people can be serious about things that are truly bothering them, this goes to a level beyond that. In my experience, younger people are far more open with their troubles with mental health. They are more likely to joke or commiserate to relieve stress and connect with each other. Mental illness is less viewed as something to be ashamed of and more as just a part of our lives. For example, in high school I could be talking to a group of people in a club, mention that I have an anxiety disorder and at least one other person will say something along the lines of "Oh yeah? Me too!" Or someone else will chime in and mention that they have severe depression, and we will all nod along in understanding or compassion. Sometimes we will discuss it a bit and maybe even make a few jokes that we can understand and relate to and sometimes we don't, and the conversation just moves on. I enjoy having those relationships and being in that kind of environment. I feel like I am understood and not judged for the cards I was dealt. It's not something to be ashamed of but accepted. A sense of community and connection is fostered. Not that it is without its downsides.

Sometimes we will not realize how serious our own afflictions are during our joking, but nothing is perfect. The good thing is that when one of us has a problem, at least a few of us can understand to some extent what is going on and what it is like. For example, one time I was supposed to give a presentation for my group to the class — we all had to do at least a some of the talking. I was chosen to do the rebuttal to the other group we were talking with, and that meant I could not prepare a statement beforehand. I knew I was not the best for this role, but somehow my group roped me into it. When the time came to give my speech, I froze at the podium in front of the entire class. I stood there for a couple of minutes as I watched the time slowly trickle away. Eventually, I ran out of the room and into the hallway, crying. I stayed out there for the rest of the class, but I was not alone.

Occasionally, someone would come out to comfort me. Some of them I knew had similar anxiety problems as me, some of them I do not know, but I believe being around people who treated mental illnesses as simply just another aspect of life helped them to be more understanding. Heck, they had more understanding than the teacher! Who told me she would talk to me for a way to get the points I lost back then never talked to me about it and just took the points away (it was an Advanced Placement class, so I was especially mad about that). When I am experiencing something with my OCD, it's comforting to know I have people to talk to that understand, either because they have it or because it has been destigmatized to them. I appreciate how far the older generations have come on mental health, but there is still more that can be done to make these topics more commonplace and understandable to the general public.

Meanwhile Breaganna was struggling with speech and language complications. She has Mixed Expressive Receptive Language Disorder (MERLD). It can make it difficult for her to process what people are saying and also difficult for her to communicate in return when she does understand. This often had me making accommodations for Brea that I wouldn't have made for Finn at the same age. When a child has a hard time expressing themselves, the default is often crying or whining. I'd watch Brea walk up to a cabinet and point as she tried to find the words to tell us what she wanted to eat. She would look at one of us and point. We would go through the cabinet guessing at one thing or another as the frustration and tears built until they burst, and she sat on the floor crying. I wanted to cry along with her.

Brea went to speech therapy without fail, but it was a slow process to teach her to speak. This added an extra thick layer of stress to a household that was already on high anxiety due to Finn's OCD and my faltering relationship with Sean.

During this time, Sean and I finally had a serious talk about where we were in our marriage. Having been nothing more than roommates for a long time, Sean and I decided everyone would be happier if we divorced. So, after twenty years of marriage, counselors, tearful discussions, and attempts to make it work, we decided we would part ways but remain friends. We truly wanted each other to have the opportunity to find happiness with someone else. However, we decided to live together for a while longer as we sorted out our finances.

I did my best to try and diffuse the building tension in the house with the kid's issues and the demise of my marriage. Meanwhile, the tension in my own chest felt ready to burst. Running was my saving grace. I could pop on my headphones and run until I felt better. I solved problems during those alone times, let out frustrations, found new ideas for my writing, and prayed.

But even this was an obstacle since I had to time the runs when Brea was in school. During the summer, it became more difficult. If Finn was stressed out, I felt bad about asking her to watch Brea. We had no family members living nearby, and Sean worked a lot of overtime. I admired his work ethic and efforts to pay down our debts, but it made finding a break tough for me. Sometimes I would even get dressed to go but then realize that my kids needed me too much for me to get a workout.

My faith didn't align with the Pentecostalism of my youth or the Catholicism that I'd embraced after my marriage to Sean, though I deeply respected both. My belief was a simple knowledge of something bigger than myself that was also part of myself. I don't believe in doctrine. I believe in love, energy (I was a physics major in college before the math brought me to tears) and directing that love and energy toward those who need it. Those thoughts of love and healing were the inhalation and exhalation of an exhausted mom running down the sidewalk mile after mile in a sea of gratitude, grief, and love. While none of those things would "fix" my problems, I didn't expect them to. Love simply changed my heart. I was grateful for all the broken, beautiful people around me and felt privileged that God had entrusted them to me. When I arrived back home from those runs, I always felt better.

One such challenge was whether to find a prescription to help Finn. For a couple of years, the subject of medication had come up. Finn didn't like the idea of it. And the OCD for which she would get the medication in the first place made it even harder for her to evaluate this issue because paranoias arose around the medication. Some were legitimate, like concerns over side effects and whether the medicine would alter her personality. There are a few people who have suicidal thoughts as a side effect. This is horrible knowledge for someone who has Harm OCD. Now they will be asked to take something that might confirm some of that paranoia that everyone has been trying to convince them isn't real. One of the Harm OCD paranoias for her was "what if I accidentally kill myself?" She would assure me she had no urge to kill herself, but the Harm OCD would have her asking, "What if I do? What if I just up and do it?" Of course, there is no using a logical argument such as, "If you don't want to kill yourself, then don't kill yourself." Harm OCD isn't interested in logic.

After yet another extensive search for therapists that would take our insurance, we found a psychiatrist not too far away. We'd gone the therapy route before, but she was reaching a point where her life was feeling unmanageable. The intrusive thoughts were back with a vengeance. Even crossing the floor could be a chore. She told me that she would sometimes have trouble crossing from one side of the room to the other.

For example, she told me of having a violent thought while touching a lamp in our living room. This meant that she had to go back to the lamp, hold on to it and think the right thought before letting go. This would work initially, but then she would get halfway across the living room and think that she wasn't paying enough attention to the right thought while holding the lamp. She made her way back across the room to hold the edge of the lampshade yet again to think the correct thought. Then she would try to make her way across the room once more. She told me this type of thing had happened at school as well and she worried people would notice and think she was weird.

Sometimes I would come into the living room late into the night and find her sitting on a certain spot on the couch, she would get up and make it through the living room and halfway into the kitchen before going back to the same spot on the sofa.

"You all right?"

"Don't ask!" she growled. "It's stupid effing OCD."

"I'm sorry," I said softly, knowing that this was one of those times when even encouraging words might be an annoyance. That's another thing that OCD robs from its targets, the very human need for comfort. OCD can render the sufferer so exhausted and irritated that even soothing words can be too much to handle. And if the person can accept kind words, other categories of OCD arises: scrupulosity, morality, and precision. *Did I thank the person appropriately for their encouragement? If I don't thank them appropriately, they will think I'm a bad person? Did they hear me say thank you? Maybe I should ask them if they heard me or say it again? They will think I'm weird. If I don't say thank you again, maybe I'm a bad person.*

### Finn says:

When you are constantly worried about doing everything right all the time, it can leave you really tense. OCD can ebb and flow with time so as my OCD thoughts and rituals would become more common, I would get more on edge and nervy. It would also make my depression and anxiety worse, and I would have periods where I had three moods: nervous, numb (at the time I thought it was happiness or contentedness), or angry.

I was angry because I knew something wasn't right, but I also thought nothing was necessarily wrong because I had always been like this, just with less intense symptoms. I had no way to express what was wrong, and the people around me couldn't tell what was wrong because it had been a fairly slow downward slope, so they didn't see the problem. The anger would come out when I was busy or when I was somewhere very noisy or lively. For example, when my family would make dinner, some-one would be making the food, at least one person would be talking, and the TV would sometimes be really loud. So, when I was already stressed because of school and my OCD's demands, it felt like a lot.

At that point, all it would take was one question directed at me to make me snap back at them, which they did not deserve, but I didn't know how to convey what was happening, so then they would get mad at me. I would just have to make an apology and/or I would get an earful about how everyone is stressed and why I should be more grateful and appreciative of my family who is doing so much for me. I do agree it is good to be grateful, and I shouldn't have snapped, but it was really hard being surrounded by people who expected anything more from me when I could barely hold on with my OCD demands and get my homework done.

This alienated me from friends and family, and yet it felt like there was nothing I could do to make the hurt go away. Even when I would try to hold it in and not make them feel bad, the anger would flow out of me like waves, so people would still detect my bad feelings while around me. Sometimes the anger would be about something they had done or something that I knew I shouldn't be angry about, so I would bite my tongue and not say anything. Other times, it was because I felt nervous about an OCD ritual I wanted to do but couldn't because other people would find it odd, so it would start out as anxiety but over time it would turn into either anger at the world for putting me in that situation, or it would be anger at myself for wanting to do my OCD rituals.

I spent a lot of time beating myself up for feeling like I had to do my rituals and for not being "normal." Then I would get mad at being mad and not enjoying life like everyone else, and the cycle continued. Sometimes I could do my OCD ritual, but then that would open the door to worry about other things, and I would be mad because I was just so tired of having to do my rituals all the time. I just wanted to live my life and not have to do things to stop worrying. That made me worry even more. Usually, the anger would just fade into sadness or numbness.

Finn was nervous when the day for her appointment came, but ready to feel better. We chose a psychiatrist this time because they could prescribe something to calm the anxiety. However, I worried about how her dad would feel about that. He firmly believed much of the problem was diet and exercise, and I believe that is part of the equation. However, OCD is not a case of melancholy that can be banished with sunlight and fresh air. And though I did not believe he was trying to reduce it to that, I also didn't feel that he'd spent as much time dealing with her meltdowns as I did, being the primary caregiver for so long. Most of all, he had not suffered with OCD like she and I had. He did not have to battle the beast and lose over and over again. He had never lain in bed with cold sweats, shaking, and panicking while trying to resist doing some inane ritual to calm the OCD. He had never looked into that abyss and thought, is this my life now?

I finally told Finn that she was eighteen and could decide for herself whether or not to tell him about the medication. No matter what, it was a minefield given the state of our strained marriage. Part of me was afraid he would try to talk her out of it or if he didn't try to talk her out of it outright, he'd tell her how many people had suicidal thoughts while on it, and she would get too afraid of it and remain too stressed out to ever deal with the OCD.

We walked into the office with its shelf of pamphlets touting the wonders of various drugs that treated everything from depression and social anxiety to bipolar disorder.

Finn and I both were a little surprised when she was told to go pee in a cup. This was a very different situation from the therapist's office with its softer decor and soothing lighting. We waited two hours past her appointment time before she was finally called back. Brea was with us and complained about being bored. Eight-year-olds don't do well in waiting rooms for two hours.

Finally, Finn was called back for her appointment. Brea and I went outside to explore the small patch of woods around the office park, but my mind was in the office with Finn. I worried she wouldn't share enough. After all, no one wants to tell someone else, therapist or not, that they've had intrusive thoughts of killing or violence, even when they know the person sitting across from them is well versed on OCD.

When Brea and I were fresh from our tromp through the forest and in the waiting room, Finn came back into the waiting room. She held a prescription for Lexapro, an antidepressant, and an official diagnosis of OCD. I already knew that, but definitive answers can have the effect of helping a person feel they are one step closer to a solution. We felt hopeful for the first time in a long while. I was never one to believe that a drug could fix everything. In fact, if it is at all possible for one to fix a problem without a drug, then, by all means, they should. But Finn's anxiety level had become debilitating.

On the way home, Finn and I talked about how she would tell her dad about the prescription. She said she didn't feel right about keeping it from him but we both knew he would have strong feelings about it. I hadn't asked her not to tell him either, as that felt underhanded, but neither did I tell her she should. I worried that he would go over all the side effects to a degree that would activate her Harm OCD and para-noia and she would continue to suffer. Again, everyone should under-stand side effects, but those with OCD tend to jump to the worst-case scenario and take it to the extreme until they become paralyzed with fear and indecision. I guessed Finn's morality OCD would demand that she tell him anyway.

That evening, as Brea and Finn were up in their rooms, I walked into the kitchen to find Sean looking as angry as I'd ever seen. At 6'7" he's already a formidable presence, when angry, it's intimidating to say the least. He was dressed and ready to go to his job at the airport where he was a lead aircraft technician. "We need to talk."

I knew what this was about and braced myself for the onslaught. The conversation was bound to be unpleasant, but I was determined that I was doing the right thing for Finn. A mother's love is a powerful force, but it can't pin OCD to the mat with a thousand hugs. "Okay."

"Finn told me she has a prescription for anti-depressants. I can't believe you went behind my back and got her a prescription without telling me. She's my daughter, and I have a right to know."

"Well, she's eighteen now, so I thought I'd leave it up to her whether or not she wanted to tell you."

"You don't have the right to do that while she's still living under my roof and using my insurance. Do you know how many guys have come back from Afghanistan and been prescribed that stuff like candy and went off and killed themselves? That shit is dangerous. Don't you think I would need to know what to look for in case she has a bad reaction to it?"

"I understand what you are saying and probably should have told you. But most of those guys that killed themselves likely already had PTSD, and you don't know that they wouldn't have killed themselves anyway."

"But I ought to know so I can watch out for her if she starts having a bad reaction."

"I'm sorry we didn't talk about it beforehand, but I don't think you understand exactly how bad her anxiety and OCD have gotten. It isn't going away, and it isn't getting any better. You aren't dealing with this as much as I am. You're at work when most of these meltdowns happen. I literally find her on the floor sobbing. Something has to give."

"I'm pissed about this!"

I stood there watching him shake with anger. I took a deep breath and tried to put myself in his position. It would hurt me terribly to be left out of the loop with something like this. At the same time, he had never experienced OCD and could not understand the torment. Even so, the fact remained that I would have been hurt if I were in his shoes.

"You're right. We should have told you beforehand."

"I'm not saying she shouldn't take it. I just think she should fully understand what she is getting into."

"Yes, but if you drive that point home too much, it will scare her so that she will be afraid to take anything at all, and she really needs help.

I'm afraid she won't even be able to continue with her schoolwork, and she will lose her scholarship. She's so stressed out with the constant vigilance that it makes attending class incredibly difficult for her. Something has to give."

"Well, I've got to get to work," he said as he gathered his lunch from the counter and car keys from the hook. "I'll have a talk with her tomorrow."

"Okay. Drive safe."

I watched him leave for work and felt that our argument was but one more nail in the coffin of a marriage that was already over.

The two of them talked the next day, and after that she became more hesitant about taking the meds. She found various excuses to put it off over the next few days. Everything from studying for her driver's test to "Well, it's late in the evening, and it might keep me up."

After a week or so, she began taking the meds, but what was supposed to be helpful soon did nothing but make things worse. She came downstairs the next morning, ghostly white with trembling hands.

"How are you feeling?"

"Horrible. I threw up last night and couldn't sleep. I'm having terrible panic attacks."

My heart sank. I didn't think she was taking a magic pill that would fix things overnight, but I never expected the side effects would be this bad.

"Well, give it some time. The nurse said it could take up to two weeks to shake off the side effects."

"Yeah, I'll stick with it, but I think it might actually be making the OCD worse."

I wanted to cry but tried to stay optimistic.

### Finn says:

When I desperately feel like I need to do a compulsion and I cannot do it, it is as if the world is falling apart. Especially when I have an intrusive thought related to Harm OCD. It feels like I'm a murderer and there is nothing I can do to fix it. I feel like I should be terrified of myself and there is no way to redemption. Most people would say "Huh? That's a weird thought," and move on, but when it happens and you have OCD, it feels like the world slows and someone has splashed freezing water over me while simultaneously shocking me with electricity. My limbs would go numb, and I felt like I couldn't breathe and there was nothing I could do to fix it, which made me worry and panic even more. I later told my therapist about this, and she told me that while I was having these episodes, I was probably either holding my breath or breathing too shallow, and I should focus on breathing when this happens. I have followed her advice and realize I hold my breath a lot, even when I am not having a panic attack.

While I was having these episodes, it felt like my mind was running a million miles an hour and the world was floating away and there was nothing I could do to stop it. My pulse would spike, and I felt helpless, like nothing could ever fix it. Moments like this dragged on. I would usually distract myself or perform my rituals to try to stop it (which is not the course of action that will fix it, but it was all I had at the time). The worst times this would happen were when I was falling asleep or early in the morning. If you can imagine this being worse. For me, at least Lexapro made these worse. Again, it is all brain chemistry. For another person with a different brain, Lexapro may have saved their life. Everyone is different.

By the fourth day she was miserable. She threw up every day, had insomnia, and the anxiety and OCD had only gotten worse. She had not even showered since she'd begun the meds.

"I have to keep my headphones in to distract myself. But I can't keep them in when I get in the shower, and I start panicking. I can't stand it. The thoughts that I'm a bad person are so much worse now.

Mom, there's something about this medication that makes the OCD harder and darker. I don't think I can stick with it."

"I understand. We'll give them a call tomorrow."

We got on an online call with the nurse. Despite our asking to speak with the doctor, we'd only been given access to the nurse. There are some very skilled LPNs out there, but we'd hoped to initially see a psychiatrist, at least on the first visit but we'd not seen one at all. I sat with Finn while she described her side effects. The nurse offered another prescription, and Finn told her that she was too scared to take anything else and asked if she could just try therapy for a while.

"We don't do that here."

Finn was pale, shaky, and vulnerable.

I looked at Finn and mouthed "May I?" as I gestured to the computer. She nodded that it was okay for me to speak to the nurse. I didn't want to take away her sense of agency. OCD does that enough as it is.

"Hi, I'm Finn's mom. Do you mean there's no one there in that office that can speak with her?"

"No, we don't do that here, and she's a grown woman and you can't make her take her meds."

This statement really frustrated me. It wasn't just a matter of toughing out the side effects until they subsided. It was making her OCD so much worse. She explained the darkness that came over her, a sense of worthlessness, and constant panicking. Although I have no doubt that this drug could be an absolute Godsend to another person with a different brain chemistry, it simply did not agree with Finn.

I took a deep breath and tried again. "Well, I don't want to make her take her meds if it's only making everything worse. She was literally crawling on the floor looking for an eyebrow hair the other day because she had a thought about Hitler, and her OCD made her believe that if she didn't find the eyebrow hair and think the right thought before dropping it again then that meant she was a Nazi. Clearly, she needs help."

"We don't do that here. Maybe you could try Emory. They offer a service where they help you find an OCD specialist in your area."

"I've already went through them, and they couldn't find a soul in our network."

She stared at me through the screen, and I stared back. We'd just gone through five days of horror with the meds, and I didn't feel that the nurse was taking us seriously.

There was nothing left to say. I clearly wasn't getting anywhere with her. "Uhm, Okay, I guess."

"All right. Have a nice day," she said before the screen went black.

Finn and I sat there as I searched for the right thing to say. My hopes were crushed.

"Mom, I could have sworn she said she'd be willing to talk to me if I wanted to." I remembered Finn telling me that on the ride home when we'd first met with the nurse, but there was no point in rehashing that now.

"Don't worry. I'll work something out. There are lots of therapists out there. I promise you if we knock on enough doors, we will find someone that can help you, and I won't stop until I find them. I promise."

I didn't realize it at the time, but many psychiatrists only write prescriptions and monitor the drug effects, while the patient must go elsewhere for actual counseling. I cannot be the only person that finds this counterintuitive and believes that there should be a better way.

I went downstairs and immediately started searching for more therapists specializing in OCD. I combed through databases and websites. I left messages and sent emails. That evening, much to my surprise, I got a call back within an hour of leaving a message with Shala Nicely, a licensed professional counselor (LPC) who specialized in treating OCD and related mental health disorders. She was all booked up for months, but she spent a lot of time on the phone with me discussing OCD and sharing how she had suffered with it as well. I was shocked and touched that she would give so much time, after-hours, on a Friday, talking to me about Finn when we weren't patients of hers, and she wasn't making a dime to talk to a frazzled mom and offer help and advice. She was both classy and kind—I vowed then to be the kind of person who would offer my time and help, such as it is, to any frightened parent once Finn and I were on the other side of this.

Shala told me about a treatment center in our area called Rogers Behavioral. They did both intensive inpatient and outpatient treatment for OCD, and she felt confident that they could help her. None of what I told her about Finn's intrusive thoughts shocked her. It was only later that evening that I realized where I had heard her name before. She had co-authored a book I had bought Finn a couple of weeks earlier: *Everyday Mindfulness for OCD: Tips Tricks, and Skills for Living Joyfully.*[3] Although Finn avoided the OCD books. I'd bought them in hopes they would help her as much as *Brain Lock* had helped me years earlier. I'd found Shala's book to be extremely practical and insightful. Eventually, Finn would read it and benefit greatly.

"You know," I told Finn, "I talked to this wonderful lady named Shala Nicely. She's a therapist who has also suffered with OCD. It just so happens that she is the co-author of one of the OCD workbooks that I bought you. Have you been reading it?"

Finn sighed before answering. "No."

"Why not?"

"Because OCD already takes so much time from me. I don't want it to take even more," she said as she twirled a string sticking out from edge of the carpet where we sat in the den.

"But it already *is* taking more of your time. At least the time you spend reading about it would be time that you spend learning how to get rid of it. You will get done with it faster if you educate yourself about it and take control. Do you want to get better?"

---

3   **See endnote 2:** Nicely, Shala and Hershfield, Jon. (2017). *Everyday Mindfulness for OCD: Tips, Tricks, and Skills for Living Joyfully.* New Harbinger Publications Inc.

"Of course, I want to get better! Do you think I don't want to get better?"

She scrunched her brows and narrowed a piercing gaze at me, seeming genuinely hurt at the idea that I would believe she wanted OCD. "I know you hate the torment that it brings you. But it might be worth exploring that there could be some subconscious motivation for not dealing with it? Like maybe you don't feel that you deserve to get better. Or maybe you think that the constant vigilance of OCD is the only thing that keeps you from committing some horrible act."

"Yes, I have thought that before."

"You think your vigilance is the only thing that keeps everyone safe?"

"Yes."

I knew that feeling well. I believed checking the door over and over kept everyone in my house from getting murdered. "With OCD, 'the only way out is through,'" I said, quoting one of my favorite Robert Frost lines.

"Yeah. I also worry that I wouldn't have anything that defines me without it."

"I understand. But there are so many wonderful things about you. You're an amazing artist and a sweet person. You talk about interesting things. Things that matter. You're courageous and aren't afraid for people to know that you are queer. You embrace who you are. That's huge! Be defined by that."

"Yeah. But I don't want to be one of those spoiled Karens who have everything so easy," she said, referring to a white, suburbanite woman who typically was spoiled and complained about everything. Extremely unfair to women actually named Karen.

I laughed out loud. "Oh, my God! Not a chance! This struggle will always be a part of who you are. You will always be able to use that as a source of strength, long after it stops owning you. You could even use it to help someone else someday who is struggling."

"I don't even want to think about that! For so long I've felt like I had to be the good kid and please everybody, do the right thing, make sure everybody is happy and make sure they are doing what they're supposed to. I'm sick of it!"

"The morality OCD blurred the lines when you were being kind, so that you didn't know if you wanted to be helpful or you had to because your OCD demanded it."

"Yes."

Another quote went through my head: *Now that you don't have to be perfect, you can be good.* It was from Steinbeck, but for now, I kept it to myself. I didn't want her to feel like I was preaching. "It's hard to know what's genuine and what's the OCD. I get that. When I had the door-checking ritual, I had to ask myself if I was wanting to check a door or window because it might really be unlocked or if OCD was just bossing me around again."

"Yeah."

"No easy answers."

"Nope."

"I'm sorry." I got up and put my arms around her. "My Finn," I said in a singsong voice, the way I always did when she was a little girl.

"My mom," she sang back.

When we are out of answers, there will still be love.

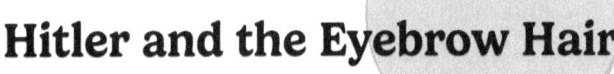

# CHAPTER 7

# Hitler and the Eyebrow Hair

Finn sat on the couch with the phone pressed against her ear. I watched a cornucopia of emotions sweep across her face as she answered one horrifying question after another.

"Yes, intrusive thoughts. Uh, huh."

She paused while the intake specialist at the Rogers Behavioral Health Institute, which Shala Nicely had recommended, asked another question.

"Well, yes, some are violent, but I don't want to hurt anybody. I'm not like that."

Before they called, I asked if she wanted me to stay or leave the room. I had a feeling they would ask some very uncomfortable questions about the specifics of the OCD as they were trying to assess the best treatment option for her. She said she wanted me to stay. She was nervous about the call. Turning eighteen is a real milestone, but scary in many ways. Suddenly, all the professionals that would have asked to speak to a parent about illnesses and insurance information can no longer ask parents. Instead, they ask a bewildered new adult who doesn't know an insurance card from a library card and can't tell a PPO from an HMO. It's scary for them.

"Yes, I've taken medication before, but it made me panic and throw up."

I can tell when they are asking her more specifics, and I can't help but mouth, "Tell them about Hitler and the eyebrow hair."

She just stares at me. OCD or not, I know she thinks her mom can be a bit much. But who could blame me? Of course, I wanted them to know just how bad things were so they could get her the help she needed and searching for an eyebrow hair in carpet fibers so you can prove to your OCD that you aren't evil like a Nazi, certainly defines someone in need of immediate mental health care.

At the end of the call, the intake specialist told Finn that a doctor would review her file, and someone would get back with her in a few days. As promised, a few days later, a nurse called back to tell Finn that her file had been reviewed and they recommended that she enter the outpatient treatment program for OCD, which would run for three to five weeks, six hours every weekday. They said that their waiting list was long, and they couldn't even provide an estimate of when a spot might open up. This was frustrating to hear because she needed help so badly. It also left us in limbo about whether to sign up for college classes in the spring. But we tried to wait it out.

The waiting proved too much. A couple of months went by with no word from Rogers. One thing was for sure, if there were that many people on a waiting list, then OCD is more prevalent than most of us realize. The intrusive thoughts began pummeling her. The bouts of crying and saying she wasn't sure she was "worthy to live" if all the images in her head were true began again. I didn't think Finn could wait any longer.

Once again, I turned to Shala to see if she could offer some advice about where to find a therapist while we waited on Rogers. She suggested we check out the International OCD Foundation[4] website. They offer lists of therapists who are Exposure and Response Prevention (ERP) Certified. This is the gold standard in OCD treatment. It involves actually having the sufferer induce the obsessive state and gives them tools and tactics to keep from ritualizing. Every time the sufferer gives in to the demands and rituals of OCD, this reinforces the rituals and habits, and the brain will repeat the process, looking for more and more assurance, digging the same harmful neural pathway deeper and deeper, and ultimately making it harder to break free. This

4   See endnote 3: This is an invaluable resource for those experiencing OCD and their caregivers as well.

process involves living with being uncomfortable and uncertain. The patient must accept the stress and panic attacks while not ritualizing either mentally or physically, as is the case with someone such as Finn deciding they must hold on to a lampshade while thinking the correct thought. It's a grueling process. Again, with OCD, the only way out is through. And oh yeah, by the way, it sucks! But freedom from such a beast isn't easy.

I called several mental health professionals listed on the OCD International website. We finally found a wonderful psychologist named Dr. Yong who owned a little Pomeranian dog. Its long tongue perpetually hung off to the side. She held it up to the screen during Finn's telehealth appointment.

"He comes with me when I see patients in my office. He's a good icebreaker," she said. We were still in the time of COVID quarantine and the one advantage this gave us was that it was now feasible for Finn to see a doctor who would have been too far away to make the drive in person every week.

Finn asked that I sit in on the first appointment. She explained her intrusive thoughts and handwashing to the doctor.

Dr. Yong explained, "I have over thirty years' experience helping patients with OCD. Many of them have Harm OCD. You should know first off that the thoughts you are having, as horrible as they seem to you, are very common with this type of OCD."

I was glad that Finn could hear this from someone other than her mom. Most people know their parents will say things to make them feel better and, right or wrong, this sometimes gives less credibility to what we say. I watched Finn's face in hopes that this would bring her a sense of relief that was stronger than what I could give.

Finn nodded and mumbled. "Good to know."

Next, Dr. Yong made a statement that was simple yet profound to someone suffering from this disorder: "Thoughts are not facts."

This may sound like a no-brainer to someone not dealing with Harm OCD, but it makes all the difference in the world to someone like Finn who is in the grip of this condition and is frightened the violent thoughts might mean she's a terrible person.

The doctor spent the rest of the session going through treatment strategies they would be employing such as (ERP) Exposure and Response Prevention and breathing techniques that she would email to Finn.

Dr. Yong also shared her strategy. "I start with the least distressing compulsions and go from there. Some doctors believe in going right for the most distressing, but I believe that can set patients up for failure. I think if you can build confidence slowly, it works out better." She went over a few things Finn could work on in the meantime.

I had real hope that Dr. Yong would be able to provide her with the tools she needed to get better. They ended the phone call with plans to meet every week. In the meantime, Finn had some assignments from the doctor.

The next day Finn came down the stairs on a mission. She held out her hands and walked toward me with purpose. "Mom, come here."

"Okay. What's up?"

"Give me your hands."

She proceeded to rub her hands over mine, then called for Brea. When Brea arrived, she rubbed her hands across the top of Brea's head. Brea gave her a strange look and walked away.

"Dr. Yong says I have to touch things I think are dirty and then not wash my hands. We're starting with things that only bother me a little."

I looked at my hands.

She laughed. "Your hands aren't any dirtier than anyone else's. It's just that normally I would wash my hands before and after touching someone's hands."

"Got it."

I felt like Finn was finally on the path to recovery, but I didn't kid myself that it would be easy.

◎

During this time, life got even more complicated in our house. It was time to tell the kids that their dad and I were getting a divorce, and we both had other people in our lives.

Sean leaned against the dresser. "So how do you want to do this?" he asked.

"I think we should tell Finn today while Brea is at school. We can explain it to Brea a little later when you have your house rented and ready to move into. If we tell Brea too soon, she might be in tears and upset all the way until you leave."

"Yeah, I thought of that, too. How do we say this, though?"

"Well, she has to have noticed that we are never affectionate and don't even talk that much. She's a very perceptive person. On some level, I think she must already know how things are. When I was a kid, my parents acted like they were breaking some big news to me when they told me about their divorce, but even at nine years old, I already knew they weren't suited for each other. In fact, I felt relieved. They were fighting constantly. People don't give kids enough credit for knowing what's going on."

"Yeah, she's a smart girl. I think it will also help if we have us, George, and Kaitlyn over for a cookout or something so that the kids can see that we support each other's relationship, and no one is angry at each other. If they see us accepting each other's new partner, then they might too."

"That's a wonderful idea. I was always so impressed that your parents had dinner at each other's house after they got divorced and everyone got along."

"All right. I'll go tell Finn to come downstairs."

Finn, Sean, and I sat at the kitchen table. I had a cup of hot tea in front of me. I needed something comforting that would also afford me a few seconds when I needed to take a sip and gather my thoughts. It was strategy tea. I invented it.

"I guess you've noticed your dad and I aren't very affectionate. We haven't been for a while and really tried to make things work, but we just can't. We truly want each other to be happy though, and we still love each other but just as friends."

Sean chimed in. "Your mom and I have just been roommates for a while now. That's why I've been sleeping in the basement. We couldn't afford two residences."

Finn seemed to take it well thus far, so I continued. "We want you to know that we both have someone in our lives that we truly care about. I've been seeing George, whom you've met before, and your dad has been seeing Kaitlyn."

"She's someone I dated when I got out of the Marine Corps before I moved to Atlanta. We got back in touch over social media when I was in Afghanistan. I'm going to be finding a new place to live. You girls and your mom will stay here."

"Okay. Yeah. I've noticed you guys weren't very huggy and all."

This was something that had bothered me for a while. I didn't want Finn to think that relationships were supposed to be as unaffectionate as mine and her dads had been. We certainly weren't enemies but neither did we represent true love.

### Finn says:

In December 2019, I came downstairs one morning, and my parents said they needed to talk to me. It was with the same tone and cadence they used if I was doing something wrong or there was something I needed to do, so I immediately worried I had done something despite me doing nothing to warrant it (at least not that I could think of). I worriedly asked if I had done something wrong, they said "no" which made me feel better, but the situation still felt so awkward and scary, so I cracked a joke, and with a smile I said, "what are you guys getting a divorce or something?" and without missing a beat my mom said "yes."

I was immediately very confused, and she explained that this had been a long time coming. They said they no longer felt love for each other romantically, and they already had other people they were seeing. They said they didn't love me or my sister any less, and that we were going to do our best to get through this. They asked me how I felt and to be perfectly honest, I felt little beyond the initial shock. They had never been very affectionate, and I had long seen the cracks forming at the seams, I just never thought it would come to this.

I was also so wrapped up in my own OCD, depression, and anxiety, I was numb when they broke the news. It didn't change how they saw me, and it felt like the rational next step. I was kind of sad, but I knew nothing was going to stop it at this point. It was like someone had thrown something else onto the problem pile I would eventually have to deal with, but now it was at the last of my list of worries. Nothing much changed at the moment and the inevitable changes felt far away. An OCD trigger found its way in from this conversation, but I could narrowly avoid it. I thought, if they weren't meant to be together, then was I meant to exist? I didn't feel that way about anyone else with divorced parents; it was only me. Looking back, I felt the same checking compulsion I felt with OCD. I didn't want to ask my parents because I was worried that would make them feel guilty for splitting up, so I eventually accepted that uncertainty and made peace with it.

Her dad continued. "We want you to know that your mom and I are going to stay friends and I'm going to rent a place nearby. You can come over any time you like. In a few weeks Kaitlyn will be in town, and we want to have a cookout here so that everyone can meet."

"Okay. I'd like to meet her."

We both gave her hugs, and she seemed fine. Though of course, that doesn't mean everything *is* fine.

She would later tell me that her own life was so fraught with stress that Sean and I divorcing wasn't something she could spend her emotional energy on. True enough. She had been struggling for a long time.

Brea was a different story.

She and I sat on the bed in my room watching cartoons together when she asked, "Why is dad sleeping downstairs?"

I doubt I'm the only parent to break out in a nervous sweat over that question. So much depends on how a parent answers it. A child's peace of mind, security, perception of their parents, and the list goes on, hinges on that one delicate answer. More than anything, we want our kids to feel secure, and it's hard to shake the feeling that we've let our children down because they even have to ask it in the first place. But when I ask myself if I'd want either of my children to someday continue on in a relationship that makes them feel lonely and sad, even after trying very hard to make it work, the answer is always "no." At any rate, I realized I couldn't wait any longer to tell her. Her dad would have a new place soon and would want to show the kids around his house.

"Do you know what divorce means?"

"No."

"Divorce is when two people who are married don't want to be in a romantic relationship anymore and decide they would be happier if they weren't together. Your dad and I are getting divorced, but we are still friends, and we still really love you. Your dad will live in a house nearby and you can see him anytime you want. You can even spend the night sometime."

"I just like to sleep here."

"You can sleep here. I just want you to know that you will still see your dad a lot. Okay?"

"Okay."

She cuddled up to me and didn't say much else that day. I wasn't even sure if she understood what had happened. Her expressive/receptive disorder made it difficult for her to process.

The next day, Sean and I were sitting at the kitchen table and talking after the kids had gone to school. Things were going as well as they could, given the circumstances.

"Kaitlyn will be in town two weekends from now. Want to do the cookout then?"

"Sure." I looked at my coffee cup and watched the steam dissipate into the air. "I told Brea about us. She seemed okay. But it's hard to tell with her. You know?"

"Yeah. I worry about that."

"Me too."

There's a strange mourning that happens at the demise of a marriage. Even when you both know you want it over with, and perhaps, should have even done it sooner, two decades is a long time. The silence hangs heavy, full of memories, emotion, and ultimately, in its own transformed way, love.

Things started moving along as well as they could. We found a divorce financial planner nearby. Brea didn't bring up the divorce again. Then a couple of weeks later, she started crying out of the blue.

"What's wrong sweetie?"

"Why do you and daddy have to get divorced? You love each other. Daddy still wants to be with you."

"Sweetie, he and I aren't like a boyfriend and girlfriend anymore," I said. Though we were married, I was trying to use terms that would make sense to her, "but we are still friends. That's all we can be. I'm sorry." My chest ached when I saw tears running down her face.

"But daddy still loves you," she said.

"Baby, I'm sorry. He doesn't. He has a girlfriend now. I have a boyfriend." My heart ached for her. I hated having to tell her there was no hope.

Sean had rented an Airbnb townhome for him, Kaitlyn, and her son, Noah, to stay while they were in town for the "meet the ex cookout." Kaitlyn and Sean were planning on living together and would also shop for rentals while they were here. I knew it would be a big change for them as well. Kaitlyn and Noah were moving out of state for the first time. They would be a long way from their hometown of Tulsa, Oklahoma.

The grill was going in the back yard, and the smell of hamburgers was making its way into the house. I was having a margarita, and the "meet the ex cookout" was underway. Kaitlyn, George, and I were in the kitchen, while Sean and Noah were outside with the grill. Kaitlyn was chopping vegetables to help with dinner when George asked her, "Don't you find this cookout to be the weirdest thing?"

"Well, yes, but I think it's really nice that everyone can get along and not make enemies out of each other."

"Oh, yeah, for sure. It's just kind of weird."

Kaitlyn laughed. "Yeah, kind of weird, but good."

We sat around the dinner table talking about hometowns, childhoods, schools, churches. Sean and Kaitlyn talked about the houses they had looked at that day, what they liked, didn't like.

Kaitlyn said, "Our favorite house was a thirty-minute drive from here, but Sean said he just couldn't be that far away from the girls."

Sean chimed in, "Yeah, I'd like for them to come over, and I want to be able to pick Brea up from school sometimes, and that will just be too far to run back and forth."

Brea seemed fine that evening, but it was hard to tell if she really was. There have been many times I've asked her about something, and she would struggle to get the words out and then say, "Never mind" or "I don't want to talk about that." When Finn was little, she didn't shut down. She was eager to tell us how she felt and didn't refrain from crying if she felt like it. But she didn't have a speech and language disorder either. She grew to develop something else entirely.

Finn was her usual friendly self at the cookout, but I knew it couldn't be easy for her either. OCD is a family disease. When a family member suffers from it, we monitor everything. We monitor the TV for something we know will be a trigger, monitoring conversations, situations, the behavior of others. Now, Sean and I were going through a divorce and there was no way this would not affect Finn, even though she said she was fine. I watched her across the dinner table, hoping she was as okay as she seemed. *It can't be this easy.* I kept waiting for the "gotcha moment." I'd seen this before, her saying she was fine and it looking for all the world to be true and then a breakdown would come later. Perhaps it was even true in her own mind for a while. We all need a Scarlett O'Hara moment from time to time: "I'll think about that tomorrow." I just wanted to be ready for when it hit.

When we were all done eating, Sean, Kaitlyn, and Noah left. Everything was strange, but that is to be expected when something that had been constant for twenty years irrevocably changes. It wasn't a bad thing, but it would take some time to feel settled inside and out.

More changes were still to come as George and I contemplated moving in together.

Navigating a relationship while dealing with kids is always difficult but add a childhood speech disorder to the mix and a heap of OCD and it's beyond challenging. George had never had any children. Though that was a part of our lives that couldn't be more dissimilar, we did share the common ground of family members with mental health struggles.

During George's almost thirty-year marriage, his wife had struggled with depression. He shared with me how he attempted to help and asked questions about what might make matters easier for her. He asked about medication and counselors when things seemed particularly bad. She told him her counseling was going well, though he admitted in hindsight that he thought she just went to a "pill mill" and didn't attempt any true therapy.

Many of those years were spent with her calmly telling him she would not grow old with him. He shared that these were not tearful rants about wanting to die but her explaining to him that she would end her life on her own terms. Her father had taken his own life in his 80s when his body began to wear out and his wife had passed.

In George's last few years of marriage, his wife repeatedly told him she would be "leaving" soon, and he needed to think about who he wanted to be with when she was gone, as she knew he was the type of person who thrived in a relationship. She laid calendars in front of him and attempted to plan her exit during a time that would be convenient for him. He tried to give her reasons to live, but she found no joy in life.

When they decided to separate, the suicide talk stopped. In fact, she began making plans to move out west and rehabilitate orphaned wolf pups, and he believed she'd found a renewed purpose. He even thought keeping her in the marriage had been depressing her. A month after the divorce was final, though, she went into the woods where she loved to trail run and ended her life.

I wondered if she might still be around if she'd had a psychologist like Finn's who took the time to really talk with her instead of just writing a prescription. Then again, perhaps a counselor somewhere tried to encourage her to deal with her deeper issues, and she simply did not want to. George said that she never shared what went on in her talks with the doctor. On the one-year anniversary of her death, we went to the woods where she'd died. George had formed some pictures of her into a pair of wreaths. In the center of each, he had written "We Remember." He located a glass-enclosed bulletin board at the trail entrance and pinned the wreaths there.

Being the person in the relationship who is always okay is a good thing on one level but exhausting on another. George understood that, perhaps better than anyone I could have dated or chosen to spend my life with. Caregivers need to talk, too, but we get so used to being the ones who are fine that when the time comes to express our own feelings, we're not even sure how. Add kids to the mix and your own needs become a point so moot it feels futile to bring them up.

I tried to explain to George what it was like to feel as if you are being pulled in several directions at once. The children had to come first. I knew in his previous marriage they simply had to make time for each other. For me, I had to meet the children's needs first, then his, then hopefully, if there was enough time left over, maybe my own. At any given time, I worry I'm letting one or more of them down. They all need something. I'm no exception—I need something too, but it's usually just time to myself or a nap that I'm after.

Still, we tried to get away now and then and go to dinner, just us.

The night after the cookout, the kids had dinner with their dad, Kaitlyn, and Noah in their rental, and George and I got to go to dinner. We sat in a lovely restaurant waiting on our food as I sipped a little Riesling and tried to shift gears from the To Do list that I hadn't finished that day.

George stared at me from across the table. "How do you feel?" he asked.

I opened my mouth to answer, but no words came out. *How do I feel? Does it matter?* "Well, I don't know."

"Right now. What are you feeling?" he asked again.

I reached inside for the answer and came up empty again. I used to feel things. Affectionate things. I was married for twenty years and for most of the last decade I'd wanted the affection and attention that the man sitting in front of me was trying to give, but now that it was here, it seemed like more than I could process. The idea of it even seemed a little . . . exhausting. I looked at him and realized that the relationship I'd wanted for so long was going to require something of me, a big something. This was another person who was going to need love and affection. Was there even enough of me? Was it even fair to drag this sweet, giving, amazing man into my world?

I decided to be honest with him. To give him an out. "I'm afraid I don't have enough to go around. You're used to just having to be there for your spouse. Sometimes I'm so tired that I feel like I don't have anything left." I was feeling that way more and more lately.

"I understand. You do a lot. You deserve someone to just look out for you and help you. I want to help you. I enjoy that kind of thing. I'm good at it."

He is. He's one of those rare souls who seems to live to serve. Our writers' organization would be at a loss without him. But wasn't that all the more reason why he needed someone who could give him more than I could? "Of course," I said, "I'll do my best to give you what you need, too, but I don't want you to end up resenting me."

"Never! You're wonderful!"

I laughed. "I don't know about all that, but I sure do love you." And I hoped this life would be enough for him. If there was one thing I noticed the more I lived, it was that the universe usually didn't give me what I wanted, it gave me what I needed. But if it did give me what I wanted—and he was it, to be sure—it wouldn't be as easy as I thought.

I couldn't decide if this blessing had shown up at the worst possible moment or the very best time. I just hoped he was ready to step into the tornado.

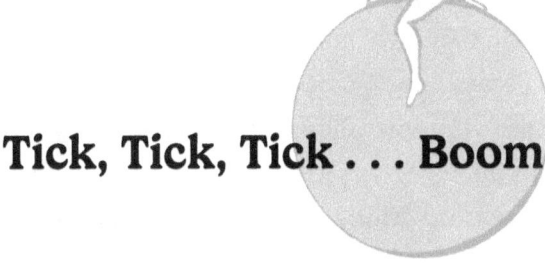

# CHAPTER 8

# Tick, Tick, Tick . . . Boom

Finn got along great with George. Neither felt that they had to conform to society's expected role for them. They were both meeting life on their own terms. They also related to the creativity in each other: though George was a writer and Finn an artist. Not long after George moved in, we decided it might be nice to take the girls to the beach for the Fourth of July weekend. It had been a rough year, and we thought a change of scenery might cheer everyone up. But right from the start, Finn was a storm cloud.

She seemed fine through the "meet the ex cookout," fine when her dad and I sat down with her to let her know what was going on, and even fine when her dad moved out. I checked in with her a few weeks after he left to ask how she was doing, and she'd told me that with so much going on with the OCD, she hadn't had the emotional energy to spend on the divorce. She gave no indication that she was having difficulty with it. Yet, as I looked in the rearview mirror as we headed south toward Florida, something was not right. When we stopped for lunch, she was grumpy.

"Grr, Brea! Watch where you're going," she groused at Brea in the parking lot of the restaurant as she nearly stumbled over her.

Brea just looked at her.

"You all right, Finn?" I asked.

"Yeah."

I tried to engage her on the trip down but got only clipped answers. When we arrived at the pizza place in St. Augustine she had always enjoyed on previous trips, she was a bundle of scary, nervous energy.

"What kind of pizza would you like, Finn?"

"I don't know."

"Well, they have meatball, pepperoni, sausage—"

"I don't know!"

"Okay. I'm sorry. Is everything all right? Did you not want pizza?"

"It's fine!"

Every word dripped with I'm-angry-and-don't-want-to-be-here.

My heart sank. It had been such a tough year. I had really believed that getting the kids out of the house would lift all our moods. Instead, it seemed to make Finn worse. I felt pressure to get the kids back on track because George was trying to do something nice for them. He sprang for a nicer condo than was necessary, drove seven hours, and was putting in some serious effort. Then again, kids are unpredictable and moody, and this is the reality of living with them. But one thing was crystal clear: this was not a vacation for me. This was just a mission to try to cheer up kids dealing with their dad moving out and ensuring George didn't get too discouraged about being a stepparent someday.

Finn's moodiness at the pizza restaurant was making everyone nervous, except Brea. She was happy to be at the beach. I asked Finn to join me on a trip to the restroom.

"Okay, so what is your deal? You're making everybody miserable with your attitude. We're doing everything we can to try and be kind and accommodating to you. Could you just give, at least a little?"

She simply stared at me; stone faced.

"Talk to me. Please."

Nothing.

"I can't help you if I don't know what's going on."

Still nothing.

"Okay. Fine. But it is not okay for you to stomp around, ruining everyone else's vacation. I know you struggle with a lot of stress, but everyone does. We're trying our best, and you're going to have to give a little, too."

The next three days were more of the same. On the Fourth of July,

I sat on the beach with George and the girls and watched fireworks going off in every direction. It was magical.

We went home without Finn ever seeming to have enjoyed her vacation. George felt deflated that his efforts seemed unnoticed, and I wanted to fix everything but couldn't.

The summer went by, and I assumed Finn had just been dealing with her OCD and stress on the trip until one day, seven months later, in the drive thru of our favorite Greek restaurant, the bomb went off—a bomb of the emotional kind.

I believe everyone, even the most enlightened among us, carries around at least one incendiary device. Many we are not indeed aware of. If we dealt with everything at once, we would go stark raving mad. So, we package those pesky little emotional, undealt with bastards into tight volatile balls and store them away until we hit just the right bump and BOOM!

The conversation began innocently enough. As we pulled into the busy drive thru, I brought up the subject of this year's upcoming vacation. "The fireworks over the ocean last year were so magical that I thought we might go see it again, so we rented another condo there. Are you looking forward to it?"

She shrugged her shoulders. "Meh."

"Would you rather go somewhere else? I don't think we can change our reservations at the condo, but if there is somewhere you might like to go for a weekend, we could look into it."

"Do you want to know why I was miserable in Saint Augustine last year? Do you?"

It all came out in such a rush that I felt like an emotional grenade had just gone off in the car with no warning.

"Um, okay, if you want to tell me."

"You didn't even ask me if I was okay with going there, and you knew that's where we had taken our family vacations. It made me miss dad. We had so many memories there. And I'm sad that people don't see me well enough to know that I don't like the same things anymore."

"I'm sorry. I didn't realize that was an issue for you. I asked you if you were doing okay with the divorce, and you said you had barely thought about it. When your dad and I sat down and talked to you, you were fine with it. When I mentioned going to Saint Augustine, you were fine with it. We told you ahead of time. Why didn't you say anything?"

"Because I didn't want to make you feel bad!" She began sobbing.

"But everyone *did* end up feeling bad. You had an attitude the entire time. Wouldn't it have been better to communicate beforehand than to get down there and be grouchy and make us pay the whole time? Do you realize how unfair it is to be angry at someone for something that you won't tell them about to begin with?"

"Now you're making me feel bad," she cried.

"I'm not trying to, and I'm sorry that you are struggling. I just want you to look at this situation and understand how much hurt and hardship could have been prevented for yourself and us if you had just communicated."

"You're making me feel like this is all my fault. It's all my fault."

I took a deep breath. "You're young and your brain isn't done developing. Hell, none of us are ever done learning what we could be doing better." I had a little emotional bomb exploding as well. Throughout the whole divorce I had been concerned that I would mismanage some aspect of the divorce and hurt the kids. Now I knew, no matter how careful, it was impossible to catch everything. Mom-guilt settled on me, heavy.

"I felt bad that dad was home alone that weekend while we were at the beach. It made me feel like I couldn't have any fun."

"Well, first of all, your dad wasn't home alone. He was working that weekend. Second, parents don't sit around stewing because their children are having fun without them. We are genuinely happy to know that our kids are enjoying themselves even if it isn't with us all the time. I promise you; your dad would not want you sitting around feeling bad. I know, for an absolute fact, that your dad loves you and would want more than anything for you to be happy at the beach. And sweetie, he isn't alone. He has a girlfriend."

"Well, she didn't move in until a couple of weeks later."

"I understand that you love your dad and were worried about him."

## *Finn says:*

Immediately after George moved in, he took us to the beach. Most people would see that as sweet or touching, but for me vacations are very stressful. You are forced together in a small space with people you already have a ton of tensions with, away from what makes you comfortable and you have to be on your best behavior the whole time. You're expected to have fun. It feels like a performance to me. I know that is how some people relax and unwind, but for me, it is the opposite. I have to prepare for the vacation and make sure I'm ready to be stressed for the next few days, and then when I get back, I have to calm down after being around people for so long.

When we left on vacation immediately after he moved in, I was super stressed, not only that but he paid for the vacation which is super sweet, but I felt like that meant two things. First, it meant he was trying to buy my affection; I know it is nice when people buy things for you, but I felt like I had to give him back my happiness. I could not be upset and sad that everything was changing at once, and I didn't know how to cope, so it made me angry that I wasn't able to be myself. Second, I felt like this meant I was not allowed to voice my opinion. I wanted to say how I felt, but I couldn't without being rude or ungrateful. I am, to be perfectly honest, a bit upset about this still because when I explained it to mom later it felt like she didn't understand. No matter how many times I told her, she would just ask why I didn't tell her to begin with. I would explain that I didn't want to be rude and make anyone feel bad. I already knew she was trying so hard, and I was trying my best to be on my best behavior, and yet I was so mad that it just seeped out of me.

I was also upset because I missed my dad, we went on vacation during a holiday that we always spent together. I just wanted to see him. He was working second shift then so it would have done no good anyway, even if I was at home. Me and dad were already stretched thin at the time. Our politics and opinions were changing, so I just felt like it was another problem I couldn't fix and didn't even have a choice in fixing. And we went to a place we always used to go to as a family. It felt like adding insult to injury. This all accumulated in me being upset, but I felt like I had no right to express it. Then I felt guilty because mom told me I was making her stressed by being stressed, and I was making George worry that I didn't like him. I do like him, and I liked him then too, I just wanted some time to work through it all. I felt like I wasn't allowed that, or I wasn't allowed to express it.

We finally picked up our souvlaki platters and were on our way home. "If you don't want to go with us to the beach this summer, you don't have to. I love you, and I'd love to have you with us, but I understand if you want some time on your own."

"I'll think about it."

"Okay. That sounds fine."

I grieved the idea of going to the beach and leaving Finn at home but having her come with us and be miserable was not a viable option. Not again.

There's no right way to do everything. We can believe that we've covered all of our bases when it comes to divorce, raising kids, treating OCD, and we can still fall short.

The point is, we care, we keep trying, and we wake up tomorrow morning and we do it all again, because we *love*.

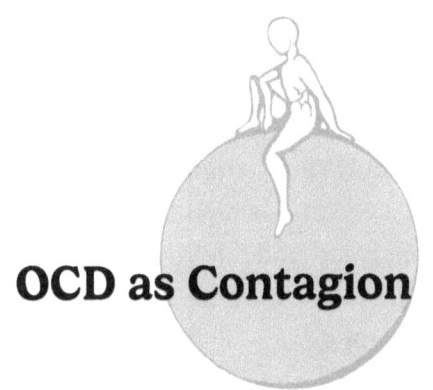

# CHAPTER 9

# OCD as Contagion

Over lunch one day, my friend Cherie told me about her tendency to worry over burning the house down. "I woke up again last night to go downstairs and check the stove. I thought I might have left one of the burners on. Wait, I probably shouldn't mention this. I don't want to make you start checking your stove now, too. You know how sometimes you aren't concerned about something until someone else mentions it?"

"Yes, I know exactly what you mean."

Later that night:

10:33 p.m. I start to drift off when I get a jolt of adrenaline. The stove! What if I left the burner on after I made dinner? I get up. I check. No flame. I head back to bed.

10:38 p.m. You only saw the flame was not on. It's a gas stove. The gas could be on. I hear my mother's voice in my head saying, "You might wake up dead." Yeah, I know, if you're dead you aren't waking up anyway, but that's something I heard as a child the first time I was given to understand that a gas leak was harmful. I get up to make sure the knob on the burner is straight up and not slightly turned and leaking.

10:44 p.m. I'm back in bed. Wired. When I left, I think the burner on the right was turned slightly to the left. *Stop that! You're being ridiculous!* Yeah, but what if the gas only kills Finn and not you? You'll have to live the rest of your life with that. Or worse, what if it kills you and Sean, after he gets home from work, but not Finn and she slowly starves to death because she doesn't know how to use the phone yet (she was still little during this particular obsession) or unlock the door to get out? I get up and check them all.

10:50 p.m. I start to drift off. Another surge of adrenaline rips through my body. My heart starts pounding harder than any time before. Check the stove! *No! This is stupid. There is absolutely no way the damn thing is on in any way whatsoever! No. I'm not going.* I hear my heart pounding in my ears. I feel like I have to go pee. I know I don't have to. For some reason that always happens when I'm having an OCD episode. Do others feel this way? Whatever. *I'm not going.* I see Finn tugging at my dead body. She has somehow survived the gas that killed the rest of us. I checked already. *Not. Going.*

I'm so tired. I just want to sleep. Maybe I could take some Tylenol PM. My head is hurting now anyway. No. It's a trap. I'd gotten into a sleep aid loop with OCD before. I flip and flop.

11:10 p.m. "Damn it!" I stomp into the kitchen once more. I stand in front of the stove being mindful of each one in hopes of not having to return. It worked that time. The door locking ritual had actually lasted longer.

Oh, the gas stove, with its myriad disasters! A killer we cook with.

Not long before Sean and I divorced, I stood in the kitchen with my heart racing as beads of sweat broke out over my forehead and scalp. My palms were freezing and sweating all at once. The glass of water in my hand slipped through my fingers. I reasserted my grip a second before it would have crashed to the ground. *Stop looking.* The man on the TV screen was being murdered. *I can't. I'm searching for something. What?* He crumpled to the ground. He was hit in the head several more times. I wanted to run from the room, but my legs felt heavy. *Just leave. Move.* My heart pounded in my ears. I kept watching. My ex-husband sat on the couch a few feet away. It didn't bother him. Why? I know what I'm looking for. A reason. I want to believe there is a good reason for this man to be killed. That someone was defending someone they loved or some such noble cause. There wasn't. Sean was fine later. He fell asleep quickly that night, while I stared at the ceiling. His brain was never "sticky."

Luckily, although George does not have OCD, he can't watch much violence because his brain is a bit sticky as well. The images bother him long after the screen goes dark. He even mentions trying to get to sleep when his mind loops some inane thing as he's hoping to wind down.

I often wonder if this is some primal mechanism meant to keep ancient man safe as night approaches. After all, we sleep in comfortable homes with deadbolts and security systems now, but it wasn't that long ago on the evolutionary timetable that we were sleeping in a cave with a sabertooth sauntering by in the darkness and if part of our brain didn't stay alert, we might not make it until morning. Perhaps there is a reason for this mental "stickiness" that we haven't yet uncovered. And just maybe, the OCD is an overreaction of this primal alert. At any rate, something has surely run amok.

Like myself, Finn has always had this problem with needing to be careful about what she watches. I recalled her being little and sobbing after accidentally seeing violence on TV. She would rock back and forth crying and telling me, "I can't stop thinking about it."

The OCD mind is often described as "sticky." It's an accurate description. There are things I've heard or watched that haunt me to this day. Watching or listening to the news can be difficult for me. I can hear a disturbing report and wake up in the middle of the night staring at the ceiling, willing myself to think of something else as cold sweat breaks out over my body. Even years later, the same scene from a movie or snippet of testimony from a murder trial might send me into a panic attack.

People can often misunderstand this tendency as well, sometimes believing you avoid things because you don't care. I had gone through this with my former mother-in-law. She'd once held up a book written by the wife of a man who had been on board United Airlines Flight 93 on 9/11 that crashed into a field near Shanksville, Pennsylvania. The man had heroically helped with the struggle to retake control of the plane from hijackers. "Have you read this book?"

"No. I don't think I could handle it."

"Well, this is real life. These people really went through something and have a remarkable story to tell. She lost her husband."

I cringed. She seemed upset that I refused to read it. I tried to explain. "It isn't that I don't care. I care too much. If I read it, I won't be able to let it go. I'll wake up at night panicking. I've read things like that and spent years losing sleep as scenes play over and over again in my head. There's nothing I can do to fix what happened." I pointed at the book. "When I was a children's advocate," I said referring to my volunteer work in family court as a (CASA), court appointed special advocate for children in foster care, "I could hear their stories because I could do something about it. There's nothing I can do to fix that."

At that moment, I realized it wasn't just the OCD that kept me from those types of books, movies, or TV shows, but also the sense of futility. Because the OCD should have continued whether or not I could help the kids I advocated for. OCD doesn't respond to logic. Never has. Along the way, OCD has a grace of teaching us something about ourselves. It taught me I'm not entertained by someone's suffering. If I'm going to take the time to hear it, then to my ears, it's always going to sound like a call to action.

To her credit, her face softened, and she said, "Yeah, it is hard to read."

In many ways though, I understand where my mother-in-law was coming from, there have been so many movies and books I've wanted to share with Finn but then realized that it might be a trigger due to violence or the subject matter. When I avoided sharing these things with her, was I enabling? Most parents would agree they don't want their children to watch excessive violence. And God knows, OCD aside, violence simply sticks with me, but there is a fine line of enabling where we protect our family members suffering with this disorder, especially those with Harm OCD specifically, to a degree that has us jumping couches like track stars over a hurdle to grab a remote when a certain commercial or news clip comes on the television to keep loved ones from being triggered by intrusive thoughts. This too can be a problem.

OCD affects the entire family. Our worlds can get smaller and smaller until the whole household is being controlled by this disorder. Those experiencing it already deal with more than their share of guilt. Sometimes, I think the residual guilt that comes from triggering someone with OCD can be just as bad. I've certainly spent time beating myself up over having mentioned something or having left something on the TV that upset Finn, but then again, we don't grow if we are protected from everything.

We can also trace our compulsions to our past. That's not to say our past gives us the disorder. It doesn't. However, it might shape the kind of, or manifestation of, compulsions we are drawn to. When I was a teenager, my dad had a tumultuous relationship with his second wife. They were in constant arguments that would often turn violent. On one of the many occasions that she locked him out of the house, he punched a hole in one of the glass panels above the knob of the door leading into the kitchen from outside. After they divorced, he left to take a job out of state, leaving my sister and me at home by ourselves. We were teenagers, and I used to have dreams that someone would stick their hand through that busted panel, get into the house, and attack us in our sleep. They easily could have. I've often wondered if this was where my door-locking compulsion came from. Probably. Years later, I drove Sean crazy with it. My former mother-in-law had even caught me checking her doors when we visited her house overnight. I explained that I'd transferred my door-locking habit to her home.

OCD isn't contagious, but it does reach out its dark tendrils and find a way to infect those around it and it is no wonder with all of the things misfiring inside the brain all at once to create this perfect storm.

Scans of the brain of a person experiencing this disorder show that several different parts of the brain are faulty. The orbitofrontal cortex associated with detection of errors and whether or not something remains rewarding—checking a door thirty times was no longer rewarding but I kept doing it—are faulty and tend to be of smaller volume than normal in imaging tests. On scans they also appear to be "overheating." To make things worse, the cingulate gyrus will then link an emotional response with the incoming error to ensure you are distraught enough to try to fix this! The caudate nucleus, deep in the brain, receives information from both these areas and sends it on to the thalamus, which often has a larger volume than normal in OCD experiencers, where it is sent out to other parts of the brain and back to the orbitofrontal cortex, which, as mentioned, is already not functioning normally.[5]

The caudate nucleus is supposed to prevent overstimulation, but it is another part of the brain that is already in dysfunction, so it does not do its job well. The devil's triangle is not a weird area of the Atlantic where ships disappear, it's in the brain of the person with OCD. And for a final whammy, as if all these things weren't enough, an area of the brain associated with planning, attention, and response inhibition tends to be thinner in the person with OCD.

There is also a form of OCD that stems from PANDAS or Pediatric Autoimmune Neuropsychiatric Disorders Associated with Streptococcal Infections. In this case a child can very suddenly develop obsessive compulsive symptoms and anxiety where there was none before the infection. I might have even wondered about this with Finn, given the illness and subsequent, serious bout with hives when she was young.

---

5   **See endnote 1:** Schwartz, Jeffrey, and Beyette, Beverly. (2016). *Brain Lock: Free Yourself from Obsessive-Compulsive Behavior: A Four-Step Self-Treatment Method to Change Your Brain Chemistry.* New York: Harper Perennial, pages 46-49

However, she'd started exhibiting symptoms before that and we certainly have obsessive compulsive disorder firmly embedded in the family history.

None of these explanations are things we can see when we meet someone though. This is why I like the example Dr. Jeffrey Schwartz, author of *Brain Lock,* uses from research done involving people with Huntington's disease, a genetic disorder that causes breakdown in the nerve cells of the brain. They were asked to sign their name repeatedly, a task that used to be easy and automatic. This simple action became something they had to consciously think about because the caudate nucleus and putamen were dying. In the case of Huntington's there were unwanted movements that they had to struggle to control. For those with OCD, unwanted thoughts must be controlled. As Schwartz puts it, "the gate gets stuck open" in both cases, but one has to do with movement, the other has to do with thought.[6]

Here again we see one of the main frustrations with mental health, with Huntington's we can see the patient make uncontrolled movements that they obviously cannot help, but we can't see what's going on in the mind of a person with OCD. It is much easier to look at the person with a mental disorder and say, "Don't think like that . . . Stop worrying . . . Give your worries to God . . . You have to take control of your thoughts." We don't usually see cancer either, yet we don't assume the cancer patient can simply tackle it themselves if they were just determined enough.

It's a wonder anyone with OCD can make it through a single day without a complete meltdown, sadly, some don't.

---

6    **See endnote 1:** Schwartz, Jeffrey, and Beyette, Beverly. (2016). *Brain Lock: Free Yourself from Obsessive-Compulsive Behavior: A Four-Step Self-Treatment Method to Change Your Brain Chemistry.* New York: Harper Perennial, pages 50–51

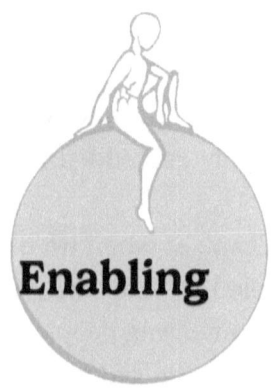

# CHAPTER 10

# Enabling

One thing is for sure, we are lucky to live in a time where information about OCD is readily available. Not only can we look things up online with just a few keystrokes, but there are also many books on the subject, though I'd yet to read many personal stories on Harm OCD specifically, which is why I felt called to write this one.

The first book I'd read about OCD many years ago was *Brain Lock*, but since then, there have been many more. Jon Herschfield's *Overcoming Harm OCD*[7] was excellent, and of course, the book he's written with Shala Nicely, *Everyday Mindfulness for OCD*,[8] was very useful. Shala's books addressed the idea of being kind to oneself as well. This was something Finn desperately needed. Dr. Yong has pointed this out many times. She even made up a game for Finn to play where she gave herself kindness cards anytime she found she was being too tough on herself.

All my research, especially on Harm OCD, leads back to the sufferer's need for reassurance and cautioned family members to avoid giving it. A person with OCD can never break out of the trap of self-doubt if they don't practice trusting themselves.

While Dr. Yong was busy noticing things, she also noticed how many times Finn mentioned coming to me for confirmation. The conversa-

---

7    **See endnote 4:** Hershfield, Jon. (2018). *Overcoming Harm OCD: Mindfulness and CBT Tools for Coping with Unwanted Violent Thoughts.* New Harbinger Publications Inc.

8    **See endnote 2:** Nicely, Shala and Hershfield, Jon. (2017). *Everyday Mindfulness for OCD: Tips, Tricks, and Skills for Living Joyfully.* New Harbinger Publications Inc.

tion with the doc was one that I realized was forthcoming. I knew Finn was asking me to confirm everything from whether she was a potential murderer to whether she should apologize to someone that she may or may not have offended (the answer is nearly always "no" because the offenses are generally contrived by OCD) and whether she might have inadvertently said something to offend them in the first place.

### Finn says:

If wringing reassurance out my friends and family were a sport, then I would be a pro athlete. Whether it be through openly asking them or watching for subtle hints, I had learned how to get what I needed to make my OCD leave me alone. In the end, this only made everything way worse, but it felt like the right call in the moment. Please, if you have OCD, don't be like me by doing these things.

Before we figured out that reassurance was not good for my OCD, I would openly ask my mom or my dad if I was being crazy or silly. They would say "yes," I would get my reassurance and go on with my day. I would also ask if I was being "stupid" by thinking certain things or I would outright tell them to tell me I was being stupid or silly or ridiculous, which doesn't help with self-esteem either, but it made me feel better about the OCD *in the moment*. This was a bandage that only temporarily fixed things.

After we learned that reassurance was bad, and they weren't supposed to give it to me even when I asked, I still found ways to get what my OCD craved. When I would ask my mom if I should feel bad about something—if she were in the same situation—or be worried about something, I would listen to her tone, watch her body language, and wording. If she said, "I shouldn't give you reassurance," then that meant I was having an OCD worry, and if it was an OCD worry, then I was probably overreacting, and I didn't need to worry about it. Which reassured me.

A big issue is that all the problems that sound ridiculous to normal people sound totally valid to me. Therefore, I can never tell what a legit worry is and what is just my OCD. I am trying my best to learn, but it is confusing.

Finn was upstairs on her telehealth call when I heard her coming down the stairs a good fifteen minutes before the call should have ended.

"Dr. Yong wants to talk to you," Finn said.

I felt like I was being called to the principal's office. "Uh, oh. Am I in trouble?" I joked. I'd learned by reading more than one OCD book that when families try to reassure their OCD loved ones, it actually makes the situation worse. We tell them they aren't murderers, they won't hurt anyone, the door is locked, they didn't offend anyone, they don't need to apologize to the random person they had a brief conversation with, etc. But this reassurance enforces the idea that they do indeed *need* the reassurance and keeps the loop going.

As a mom, the idea of not reassuring your child when they are in tears is painful and goes against every instinct a parent has. I had considered stopping the reassurances all together and had avoided it a few times, telling Finn that she already knew the answer. OCD was just pushing her to seek reassurance, and I didn't think I was helping her by giving it. However, I didn't know if her psyche was at a place where I could stop that kind of thing outright.

I walked up the stairs to Finn's room, made my way past a pile of dirty clothes, and braced myself as I sat down, and she handed me the phone. There was Dr. Yong's smiling face on the screen, waiting to tell me that my reassurances were a problem. And she did.

"Finn tells me she comes to you for reassurance when she is struggling with her OCD, and I just want to ask that you avoid reassuring her. She has to learn to live with uncertainty, and the reassurances are actually making it worse."

"Right. I've been reading that in the various books I've ordered."

"It can be really tough to avoid reassuring a child when they are upset, I know, but you can listen and encourage. You just have to avoid concrete reassurances."

"Yeah, it's pretty obvious when she's wanting that kind of reassurance. I'll avoid it from now on."

"This will really help her progress."

I left them to the rest of their session and practiced in my mind what I might say to her next time she asked if she were a murderer, or if something was morally wrong or any other number of things. This was going to take some reprogramming on my part. Parents live to reassure.

The next day Finn came downstairs looking worried but also had that smile that said I'm-about-to-ask-you-something-that-I-know-good-and-well-I-shouldn't.

"Okay, so I know this might be an OCD question, but I don't really feel like hanging out with my friends tonight. Does that make me a bad person?"

I started to answer ten different ways, and it got more complicated than you might think. I couldn't tell her my opinion directly, but could I say what I'd done in a previous situation? Could I say that we all just feel like relaxing alone sometimes? Will she search for a "reassurance" answer in anything I say? OCD is a seeker; if an answer isn't given directly, it will seek answers in facial expressions or body language. Instead of doing any of those things, I smiled and said, "You know I can't answer that, but I love you so much and believe that you can be okay without me answering."

She made an anguished sound as she crossed her arms on the kitchen table and laid her head on top of them.

The new phrase in our house became, "I know this might be an OCD question, but . . ." and then she would launch into a variety of scenarios:

"When I was washing the dishes, I scratched the side of my nose, do I need to rewash all those dishes?"

"I'm out of hand soap, so I washed my hands with shower gel, but I don't think it counts. Does it count? I mean, it's a different kind of soap. I think they aren't really clean. I've been washing them upstairs in my bathroom then coming down here to wash them with the regular hand soap. Should I be doing that?"

"If Brea falls asleep on the couch and her face is turned toward the cushion, is she still able to breathe? I checked, but I'm not sure."

"If I'm playing a game where there are Greek gods that I'm battling, and when we all die in real life, if it turns out to be true that the whole Greek god religion is really a thing, will I then be doomed to their wrath?"

"If I go to bed, and my dirty feet are all over the bottom half of my mattress while I sleep, and I then touch that part of my mattress, do I need to go wash my hands again?"

"If I kind of like a villain in a game, does that make me a villain?"

And of course, the BIG question, "If I have flashes of thoughts about murder, does that make me a murderer?"

I had been terrified of the day Dr. Yong would confront me about the reassurance. Every instinct most mothers have is to reassure and soothe. When that was taken away, it went against biology, evolution, God-given instinct, or any other way one sees that grand responsibility called motherhood. I'm sure it's no different for a father watching their children suffer.

As hard as holding back that reassurance was, it would teach her to eventually untangle the assurance trap that she, by way of OCD, had put herself in. OCD had systematically taken things from her: peace, socialization, trust, and a whole host of other things, both obvious and covert, but I never expected the next thing that OCD would conspire to take from her: *me.*

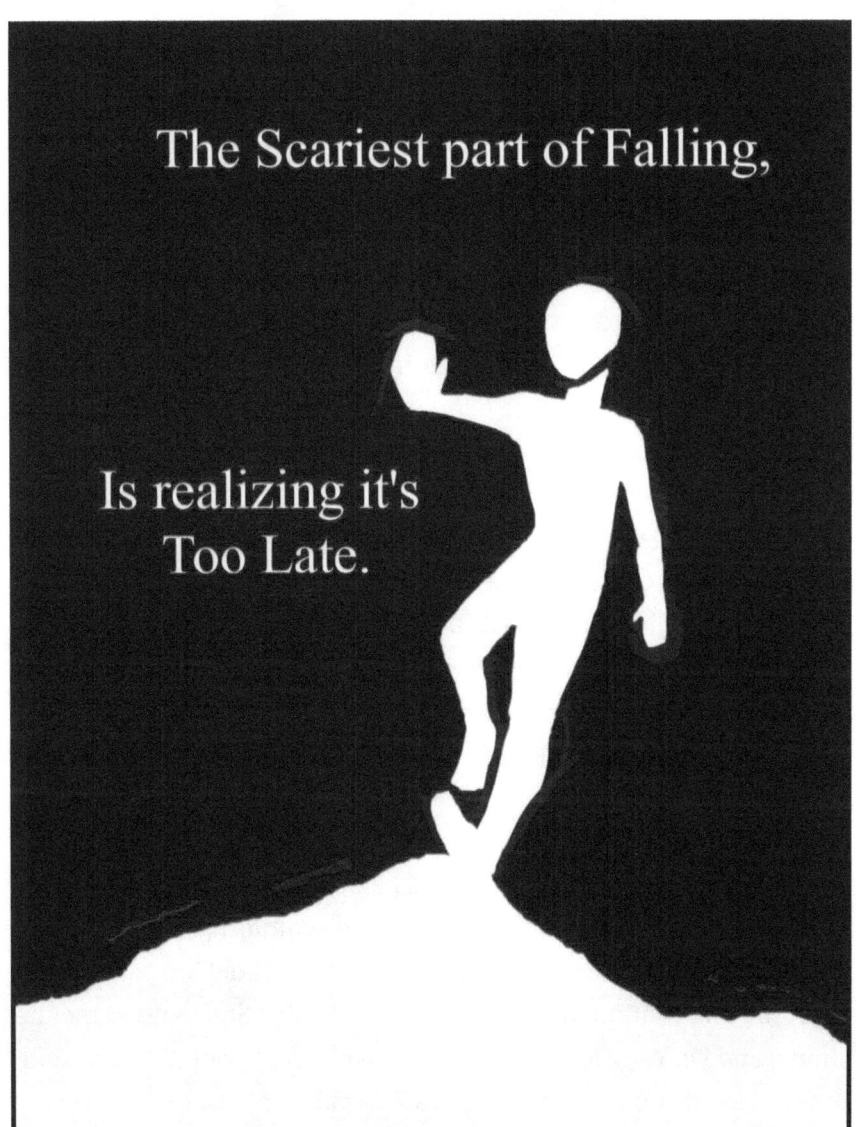

The Scariest part of Falling,

Is realizing it's
Too Late.

Illustration by Finn Conrey

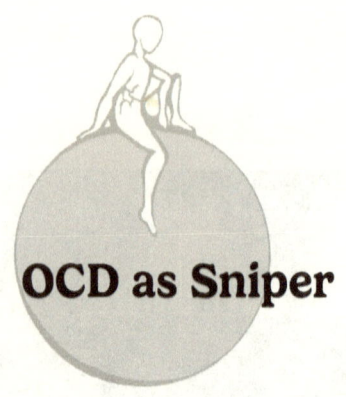

# CHAPTER 11

# OCD as Sniper

Finn continued her meetings with Dr. Yong, and sometimes during those meetings I heard wailing coming from Finn's room above the office where I worked. It called to mind old folk tales of banshees whose cries they could hear echoing through the ancient forests of Ireland, where much of Finn's heritage could be found. These wails made my chest ache as I sat downstairs, saying a prayer for her. I was sure they were in the thick of Exposure and Response Prevention therapy (ERP), where Finn induced the thought that makes her want to ritualize and seek assurance. I'd been there before, trying not to check a door for the twentieth time, trying not to reread the same sentence repeatedly, and the list goes on. It's "hell and hellacious hell" as my OCD-ridden grandfather would say, though he never knew that was what had ailed him.

Finn would later tell me this was when they'd began reading "scripts" of harm scenarios that she'd been avoiding. The script forced the brain to learn to be comfortable with discomfort. Toward the end of one such therapy session, a red-eyed, puffy-faced, Finn came down to get me and motioned for me to come upstairs. She handed me the phone, and Dr. Yong looked back at me with great sympathy and said, "I hate leaving a patient in a destressed state like this. I'm all booked up today but would be willing to talk to Finn during my lunch hour but will have to eat while we talk. I just really don't want to leave her like this all week. But Finn wanted to ask first, since you all are using your HSA for these appointments."

"Of course, by all means, go ahead. It's very nice of you to work through your lunch break."

"Well, she's really having a tough time. We knew this could happen once we started working on the Exposure and Response Prevention therapy," she said. It was just as I'd thought. She had taken Finn into some of her most upsetting compulsions—intrusive thoughts—and had her practicing not ritualizing in her head via counting, mentally repeating a phrase, reassuring herself until she felt better, or physically ritualizing by arranging things a certain way or scratching an arm a certain number of times to ensure a loved one didn't die, etc.

Finn disconnected the call with Dr. Yong and railed against OCD as tears ran down her face. "I don't understand what she expects me to do! If I just let the thoughts come, then that's like saying that I'm good with them, and I'm not okay with them, but she wants me to be okay with them. If I am, then I don't deserve to live. How can I be okay with murder?"

"No one is asking you to be okay with murder. She just wants you to train your brain to stop reacting as if it is saying something real. That gives the OCD power and validation. You're digging that little neural pathway even deeper and making it harder to stop."

"I don't understand!"

I took a deep breath and began again. "If you let the OCD play in your head and stop responding, it eventually shrugs its shoulders and leaves because it isn't getting a response out of you anymore. Every time you respond with ritual, it gets validation and keeps coming back for more and more validation. It's never enough. You stop the loop by refusing to respond."

"But that means I'm okay with murder!"

"No. It means you stop acting as if it *is* murder because it isn't. It's just a thought, not a thing."

Finn and her doctor talked again that day, and she did seem better afterwards but didn't want to talk about it later, and I didn't push.

One of the cruelest things about OCD, among its myriad of horrors, is that it tends to make a person's world smaller and smaller. Many people who suffer from it avoid social situations, just as Finn did.

However, Finn found some friends who would play a favorite video game together over a group chat. I was beyond thrilled that Finn had a group to interact with. However, a person who ran one of the game's social media pages reposted something from a fan that might have been considered morally objectionable. This sent Finn into an OCD morality tailspin that lasted for several agonizing weeks while she wrestled with the idea of whether she should stop playing the game entirely, which also meant the lifeline of socialization would be taken from her.

I was angry at OCD for trying to take this away. I'd watched her go without socializing and suffer the consequences of isolation for so long. Not having friends chipped away at her self-esteem and mental health.

We went for a walk around the neighborhood on a crisp fall day. I was glad to have Finn out in the fresh air, but I was even happier to be spending some one-on-one time with her while Brea was in school. Brea was eight and didn't respond well when she noticed me trying to spend quality time with her big sis. I was also happy that Finn was walking outside instead of pacing in her room. She had been complaining more and more about her knees aching. The pacing back and forth had her pivoting to go to the other side of the room. I suspected this pivoting over and over again on the carpeted floor was wrecking her knees.

While we walked and talked, we got back around to the topic of her game. She said, "I think the right thing to do would be to stop playing it, but I really love this game. It's one of the few joys I have in life anymore."

"Then keep playing it. Don't let OCD take this from you. It's taken enough already!" I wasn't angry at her, but I could feel myself getting angry that her mental wiring wouldn't allow her happiness.

"But it's morally wrong of me to keep playing a game that condones such thing."

I wasn't supposed to weigh in on OCD matters. "This is just a gray

area, and you need to let it go. Don't condemn an entire gaming fran-
chise over one repost on social media. That isn't fair to all the people
who worked so hard to make this game a reality. There is nothing morally questionable in the game. This is just *one* repost. It is unfair of you
to do this to yourself or them."

"Yeah, but—"

"What did Dr. Yong say about it."

"She said that I should write an email to the company if I feel that
strongly about it."

"That's a good idea. It's good to make your voice heard. Whether or
not it changes anything you will always know you spoke up."

"Yeah, but I probably need to stop playing the game, too."

"I disagree. Life is full of gray areas. I heard a story about this couple
who had been together for many years, got married, and then found
out that they were half brother and sister. They'd been adopted to
separate families and never dreamed that they would turn out to be
siblings. They agonized over it for a very long time before deciding that
since they hadn't planned on having children anyway, they would just
stay together. I'm not saying they should or shouldn't. All I'm saying is
that I'm not going to judge them for that. I believe this is a gray area.
They had no idea they shared DNA. It isn't fair to them."

"No. It's wrong. That's just wrong."

"Okay. You're entitled to feel that way. I'm just saying there is so
much gray area in the world and until you accept that, you will be
stuck in this trap of scrupulosity that OCD demands."

I didn't think much more about it that evening. The next day
she came down for dinner barely speaking, head down, eyebrows
drawn together. I knew the look and feared it. We had dinner and she
remained quiet throughout. George got up to do the dishes, which he
did most of the time as he noticed that is usually when Finn is in the
mood to talk to me.

I took a deep breath and asked Finn, "Are you okay?"

"Just OCD stuff."

"I'm sorry. Do you want to talk about it?"

She crossed her arms over her chest and burst into tears. "I can't trust you anymore."

"What? Why?"

"Because I count on you to know what is morally right when I can't, when my OCD confuses me. Now you said that it's okay for the brother and sister to be together and it's wrong. It's just wrong, and I can't trust you anymore." She started sobbing so hard she could barely be understood.

I looked a few feet into the living room area where Brea was watching TV. She had heard the sobbing and turned to stare at her sister.

My heart broke as I was hit with the realization that OCD was not only taking away the things she enjoyed, but now it was picking off people that she loved as surely as a sniper on a hill. It was aiming for me now. And I was pissed. I'd lost countless hours of sleep looking out for her. I'd worried and anguished my way through many days and nights, and now OCD had the audacity to judge and banish me.

It was painful to say the least. I didn't deserve this. Luckily, I was able to separate Finn from the OCD. This wasn't her fault. But it did go to show that she had to work hard and put in the time to get better because this thing was looking to isolate her and knock off anything and anyone that couldn't pass its codes of rigidity and scrupulous morality. I realized now that it would continue until nothing and no one was left. Not even Finn.

Finn's sobbing continued and Brea walked over. "I'm sorry you're sad."

"Thank you, Brea," Finn choked out between sobs.

"Maybe a stuffed animal will make you feel better. Maybe I can buy you a teddy bear. Will that make you feel better?"

"I don't think so but thank you for asking."

"Okay," Brea murmured before going back into the living room to watch TV again.

I spent the next hour talking to Finn, and she started in again with the idea that if she was capable of horrible things then she didn't deserve to live.

"Finn, that isn't true. No one can ever know anything one hundred percent every time."

"I have to know. And if it's true, I don't deserve to live. We have the death penalty for people who kill. We believe those people shouldn't live. How do I know if I deserve to live?"

"Stop it. Of course, you deserve to live. Your OCD is just messing with you, and it's never going to get enough. There's no such thing as enough assurance. That's why you need to do your workbooks when you start feeling this way. Don't sit around and feed the beast and ask the same questions that get you nowhere."

We talked in the same circles, and finally, Finn calmed down a little and went back upstairs to her room to pace. Once again, we heard the footsteps overhead. Pacing out a cadence of fear, confusion, and anger.

I put Brea to bed and came back down to talk to George. I found him at his desk. The house was quiet, and sorrow settled on me heavily.

"How's she doing?" he asked.

No need to clarify. Of course, he meant Finn. She'd been sobbing just a few feet away while he did the dishes. "Same as always." I sat down in the chair across from him and rubbed my eyes. I'd run marathons that left me feeling less depleted than dealing with OCD.

He propped his elbow on the desk, put his chin on his palm, and looked at me. "I'm sorry."

"Thanks. It really hurt me when she told me she can't trust me anymore. That was rough."

"Yeah, I heard."

"I know. I'm sorry." Probably not what he had pictured when he moved in with us.

"That's okay. I'm here to help you. We're in this together."

"Thank you." Once again, I marveled at his ability to jump into my household—at the worst possible time he could have jumped in—without running for the hills. "Luckily, I'm able to separate the OCD from her. She isn't trying to hurt me. I know that, but still, having someone that you've given up so much for, and love so much, tell you that they can't trust you anymore, like you are a villain. It just hurts so much."

"I know."

I thought back again to the tearful walk through the library to search for something to help myself when I was struggling with OCD. She must have wanted to get better, but sometimes I feared she was afraid to. She believed constant vigilance was needed lest she relax for one moment and have some heinous action break through.

"I can't think about it anymore."

George and I sat and watched a few episodes of a funny sitcom to get my mind off it. I would be forever grateful to have someone like him and hoped that our relationship would bring him as many good days in our family as gloomy ones. Honestly, I wasn't sure it could.

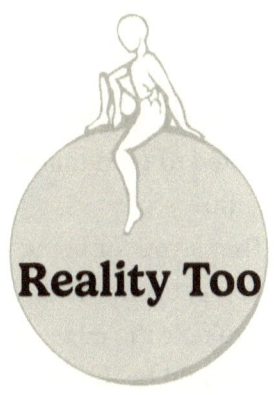

# CHAPTER 12

# Reality Too

Dr. Yong continued counseling Finn throughout the fall. She and Finn worked well together. They had begun the Exposure and Response Prevention (ERP) therapy, but many times Finn would have a breakdown during the process. Finn came downstairs during one of her sessions to let me know that Dr. Yong wanted to speak to me again. Like last time, I spoke with Dr. Yong via telehealth. The pandemic was still raging and all visits that could be done remotely were. Finn had yet to meet Dr. Yong in person.

Finn handed me her phone. "Hi, Ms. Conrey. Finn wanted me to speak with you and let you know what is going on. As you know, Finn and I have been using Exposure and Response Prevention to treat her OCD, and we aren't making much progress because her anxiety level is just too high. I believe if we could get that down a little, it would free Finn up to make some real progress with therapy, but as it stands, her anxiety is making progress almost impossible."

"Right. I can see that."

"Medication isn't my first go to. Many people can tackle this without being medicated. However, sometimes medication can be helpful to get a patient to a point of being able to implement their therapy more effectively. She's explained to me that she has had bad experiences with medication in the past."

"Yes, and I can't blame her for feeling that way. The medication really did a number on her last time."

"Right, and I want to address that. I have a colleague that I believe can help her. I've explained to Finn that I can work with this psychiatrist to explain to him the issues she's having and make sure he understands how much she struggled with the medication last time. I've also explained to Finn that she will need to sign a waiver for me to speak with him."

"Thank you for being willing to do that. I also believe that if some-one can get better without medication they should. But having some-thing to take the edge off long enough to make some progress sounds like it would be the best thing for her right now. Would you be willing to speak with her father if he has some questions? I know he has some concerns about medications. He's a veteran, and he's worried that so many of his fellow veterans returning from combat were on antide-pressants when they committed suicide. Of course, many of them had PTSD and may well have taken their lives regardless, but this is some-thing that is scary for him."

"Yes, of course. I'd be happy to answer his questions," she said.

"Thank you so much. He may not even need it, but it would be great to offer that as an option if he gets worried about it again."

Later, Finn told me that Dr. Yong helped her compose an email to the psychiatrist. I appreciated that she was having Finn be an active participant in her recovery instead of sitting on the sidelines and hav-ing others arrange and manage it.

It would still be several weeks before the psychiatrist, Dr. Landers, could see her and arrange a prescription for Finn. In the meantime, there were breakdowns and much reassurance seeking. I looked toward her appointment with the hope that it could relieve some of the pressure enough to make some progress with the therapy. Her dad and I also feared that without some relief from her anxiety, Finn would lose her scholarship, which paid ninety percent of her tuition.

### Finn says:

While waiting on my appointment with Dr. Landers, I really struggled with the intrusive thoughts, including the prayers rit-uals. Looking back, I realize I carried the obsessive prayer ritual from Christian school to public high school and finally to my first year of college, in all about 5 years because my first year of college was also my last year of high school because of dual enrollment. When I would eat lunch on campus, sometimes I would have intrusive thoughts, and I would have to have a good thought before I could stand up or throw my trash away or leave my class. This would lead to a lot of awkward moments where I would try to leave but at the last moment, when my body still had contact with the object, I would have a bad thought and not have enough time for a good thought before the object left my hand, so I would walk back, awkwardly touch whatever the item was while trying to look as natural as I could (which did not really work), and then I could leave. It was always extra fun when I was running late or in a crowded area where I knew a lot of people were watching me.

This would even occur when I hugged my family, I would have to have a good thought before I let go, which led to some very awkward situations, and eventually I had to tell my mom what was happening. I have broken a lot of that habit recently. Occasionally, I slip back into it, but now that I have better tools to deal with it, I struggle with it far less.

About a year after my OCD about praying faded away, I developed OCD about other things. Mainly I got invasive thoughts about being a murderer or a pedophile, so I prayed to figure out what was happening. I had no clue which thoughts meant something, and which ones did not. One time while I was praying, I breathed in deeply and got a lighter feeling in my chest as I asked God to give me a sign. I took that as a sign that I wasn't an evil person. Then whenever I would have invasive thoughts, I would run off somewhere private, pray, ask God a question, take a deep breath, and decided that whichever follow-up thought made me feel lighter was God's answer. If I didn't feel especially lighter after an answer, I would try again. I would also try again if the answer wasn't what I wanted, and

I would chalk up the first answer to human error. Sometimes I would take deeper breaths to get a lighter feeling while I was trying to get the answer I wanted.

I sort of knew I was lying to myself, but to get some relief I kept going through the ritual, I also thought if it got me the "true answer" or "God's approval" this process was worth it. Eventually, I began to worry and overthink things, and I had to pray longer and longer to get my reassurance. This behavior stopped when I stopped praying daily. I had a fallout with my faith and no longer wanted to pray as I had done. I am still spiritual, but not religious. Since I was no longer praying, the problem cleared itself up. I found other rituals to take the place of that though, so it wasn't really a way out.

Her anxiety and OCD made it hard for her to concentrate. In addition, the scrupulosity with her assignments and instructions made school very stressful. She often procrastinated because she knew once she started an assignment the urge to make it perfect would kick in and take up all her time. Therefore, she didn't have the usual dread of work that students get but instead she experienced the added pressure of knowing OCD would have her pouring over details and getting stuck in the loop of perfection. Group projects were particularly difficult as her OCD demanded that she find a way to keep everyone happy, even though she knew there was no way to do so.

However, sometimes OCD had a secondary effect. I knew I had to remember that her problems weren't always related to her condition, especially on the night she woke me at 3:00 a.m. with loud knocking on my bedroom door, I stumbled from my room worried something awful had happened but mostly feeling sure it was just more OCD.

I opened the door to find Finn saying, "Please don't be mad at me," before I had the chance to even ask what was wrong.

"I'm not mad," I said as I squinted through dried-out contact lenses. "What's wrong?"

"I put off my project because I just want to enjoy my life. I'm sick of worrying about school and always having to be the responsible one. Anyway, the deadline is midnight, and I didn't get my project done. Now I'm afraid it's too late, and I'm exhausted. I don't think I can stay up any longer. I'm so tired."

"So, you're going to lose your scholarship because you don't want to do your work?"

"Please don't be mad."

"I'm not mad. But you need to get in there and do your project. I know you're having a hard time, but you can't just mess around and refuse to do your work."

"Okay. Sorry." She turned around and shuffled into her room to finish her late assignment, because sometimes the problem isn't OCD. Sometimes, it's just a college student who doesn't feel like completing her assignments.

That's reality, too.

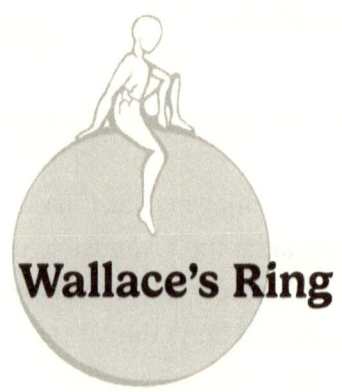

# CHAPTER 13

# Wallace's Ring

I looked at my engagement ring as I *breathed in and breathed out.*
The ring belonged to a man named Wallace and the woman he was to
marry, Ina. George just told me the doctor thinks he has COVID-19. *It
comes from a bat.* "Does this mean you'll develop sonar now?" I asked.

"What?"

"Well, you know, it's a virus from a bat. Spider-Man got his powers
from a spider. So, it stands to reason . . ."

"But I'm not blind. What good would sonar do me?" he asked as
fevered chills moved through him like a wave.

"True."

He put his hand to his chest and tested his lungs. He breathed in.
He breathed out. This was long before the vaccine was available.

I tried to keep things light. The chills he described were strange.
They started at his waist and radiated up his back and shoulders and
out into his arms. His whole body twitched when they started. He
was being shaken from the inside as his body sensed the invader and
demanded that every cell heat up to fight this beast. Though the girls
were in the house with us they remained unaffected by it. So far, I
wasn't either.

We went back home to wait for lab results as his fever rages for
seven more days. I went on the internet to look up the mortality rate
for men in their fifties with COVID-19. *Breathe,* I said to myself by the
glow of my laptop.

He'd always been a doer and being this sick meant I had to *make* him go to bed. He laid down in the cool, dark room.

"I feel bad that I'm not helping you around the house," he said.

"Oh, for goodness' sake. Stop it. You're sick. You've had a fever for seven straight days. Get some sleep." I pulled the covers up to his chest and checked his temperature one more time. The fever reducer isn't doing much for him tonight. I didn't say so, but I was afraid to go to sleep. I wanted to just stay there and listen to him breathe. He swore to me it wasn't in his chest.

*He's going to be fine. Breathe.*

I sat down on the bed beside him and looked down at my engagement ring. It's over a hundred years old. It was first given to George's grandmother, Ina, during the 1918 Spanish flu pandemic by a man named Wallace. But Wallace succumbed to the flu before they could marry. No one had worn it since, until now.

On a beach in St. Augustine, George got down on one knee as he put the ring on my finger and we became engaged with Wallace's ring, a full one hundred years after Wallace asked Ina, the love of his life, to marry him during the Spanish flu outbreak. We've both been married before and second chances are a gift: a second chance at love, a second chance to redeem a ring that's never made it to an altar before. I got down on one knee in the sand as well. I wanted to be where he was. I laid my head on his shoulder and listened as the waves rolled in from the Atlantic as I breathed in and breathed out.

He looked rough. I didn't want to leave the room. "What else can I get you?" I asked.

"Just come talk to me," he said with a voice made shaky with chills. He breathed in. He breathed out.

I walked over and sat next to him on the bed. I brushed his hair back and said, "I love you." He was asleep before I could say another word.

I sat for a while, listening to him breathe.

I mentioned the ring's history to a friend, and she looked at me with absolute dread. "I don't know about *that*," she said, pointing to the ring as if it belongs to the Grim Reaper himself. "I'm not a superstitious person, but that would scare even me."

At the time, George didn't have the virus, but we got engaged knowing it was a very real possibility for either of us. So why in the world would we tempt fate with such a ring?

We believe in fate, but how we choose to see that fate greatly depends on how we view our world. Perhaps the timing wasn't bad at all. Perhaps it was just right. Maybe Ina and Wallace stand just on the other side of the veil as they watch their ring come full circle to our modern-day pandemic and rejoice that it gets to have a happy ending.

Faith follows this ring, courage, hope, and love. It's the same thing that brings doctors and nurses into the hospitals, risking their own health to care for the sick and dying. It's a type of faith that their efforts are never in vain, that they continued to treat patients knowing they might well catch it themselves. They moved forward knowing they might not see the journey's end but believing what they did right then mattered and still does. My fiancé and I both have past relationships but have the faith to try again, just as Ina had to. Faith doesn't shut away Wallace's ring in a drawer.

I laid my head on his chest and listened. His breath is faster than mine but not labored. On the ninth day his symptoms subsided. He recovered. Miraculously, I was also well—just like Ina . . .

I Breathe in. Breathed out. It was my own breath I listened for. He was eleven days recovered, but I've got fever, chills, headache, and a cough that brought a tearing sensation to my chest. Still, I wouldn't be parted with my faith or my ring.

Four days later, I walked outside, took a deep breath, and gave thanks to be well. I looked down at my hand, to the antique ring somehow now redeemed.

# CHAPTER 14

# My Neighbor's Keeper

I laced up my well-worn running shoes, put my headphones around my neck, and made my way out the door. The leaves clinging to the trees and blowing across the driveway were gold, red, and orange. My favorite time of year. Finn's anxiety level was high. I never knew when it was going to bubble over. She was always worth the effort, and I never resented her. But sometimes, I felt wrung out. There have been so many times when it might have been beneficial to let my emotions out, but a level of numbness settled over me. That wasn't always a bad thing.

We can't all be having a meltdown at once, but there were odd times of running down the road and feeling . . . fragmented, like there were pieces of me lying here and there but there was no time to stop, figure out where they went, or glue them back into place. When someone needed something, I felt as if I sorted through those pieces, looking for the one they needed and handed it to them. There is a reason we often refer to a state of mental and emotional health as "feeling whole."

I'd learned many years ago that crying fixed nothing. At least for me, it didn't seem worth the effort. We cry, make ourselves feel powerless, drag someone else into our misery, and walk away with absolutely nothing fixed. Seemed pointless to me.

Nonetheless, I'd contacted Finn's therapist about scheduling a session for me so I would know better how to handle my daughter's situation, but she felt it would be a conflict of interest to speak with both of us. Other than that, I hadn't pursued counseling solely for myself. It would've just added another layer of stress because I didn't know where I would fit it in. I already struggled to find time during the day for basic things like going for a run, showering, or even slowing down to get a glass of water or use the bathroom. Besides editing part time, I was also continuing my own writing, including writing a blog about living with OCD, and finishing up a degree online.

I cranked up the music in my headphones and contemplated the changes in my life. After we'd gotten engaged, George had moved in. We'd been together for ten months and had known each other for twelve years, but still, it was a tremendous change. Everyone, no matter how kind, generous, and giving—and he was all those things—had frustrations, habits, wants, and needs. I already had my plate full dealing the girls. In many ways, I felt as if I were being crushed. Even a great relationship couldn't just simply be enjoyed. As any parent knows, you must consider your kids' wellbeing first. If their needs can line up with what you want, great, but the first thought couldn't simply be that I wanted this because I wanted this. Those days were long gone.

I contemplated how George could enjoy things more because he didn't have kids. He could be in love in more of the sense that we are when we are younger. I worried because it was obvious, I couldn't do that. He would believe he was missing something. I tried to show him just how much I care because I knew, from his perspective, I must've always had something on my mind other than us. Then I got a little angry at the expectation placed on me, and I felt I was crumbling beneath the weight of it. *Do all mothers in new relationships feel this way? Where's the joy?*

It was nice to have someone to help me day to day, but most of all, I loved him. There was a time when romantic love trumped everything. I both loathed and missed those days. I never liked being ruled by my emotions, but I missed feeling excited about a relationship instead of being exhausted by it. I reminded myself that I didn't have kids back then, either. From the first time I contemplated living with him, I worried about the effect his moving in would have on Finn and Brea. No matter how helpful someone is, and no matter the fact that the kids knew and liked him, it would still be a stressor to have someone new in the house.

During those days, it was hard to feel anything, and I went right back to worrying that I wouldn't have enough to give.

Halfway out of my neighborhood, I encountered my friend Deanna, who was out walking her dog. She informed me of an old classmate of Finn's who'd taken her own life. As a mom of a child with OCD, my first thought was, *what if she'd had Harm OCD and believed that she was doing the world a favor by taking herself out of it? What if she had no idea it was OCD and believed that it destined her to kill?* Of course, I didn't know if any of this was true for this teenager. But I was absolutely certain that there have been individuals throughout time who've had Harm OCD and believed killing themselves was the kindest thing they could do for this world. When I was younger, I had no idea what Harm OCD was. I didn't grow up with the internet. If I had, would I have even known what to search for? I'm not even sure someone *today* would know the violent thoughts could be part of OCD. This is a disorder that has been so cliched, it might never cross their mind that violent repeating thoughts might be part of it. The OCD would have likely made me paranoid someone would see my search box about murderous thoughts, anyway. OCD presents one trap after another to keep sufferers from help.

I asked, "Was she depressed?"

"I don't know. The family isn't saying much."

"Sometimes I get terrified for Finn. She has a form of OCD called Harm OCD. She sees flashes of herself doing violent things, killing . . . I had it too when I was younger. Hers actually seems to be worse than mine. It's terrifying." I tell her how Finn says to me, "'If the images I see in my head are true, then I don't deserve to live.' It scares the hell out of me." Tears started running down my face. Pointless tears. They wouldn't change anything.

"Oh, I'm sorry." She started crying as well and made a gesture like she wanted to hug me, but the pandemic was going on. Perhaps knowing we'd both already had the virus helped to make her decision. Perhaps the very human urge to comfort someone in distress, another mom who you can deeply identify with trumped the risk. Either way, she embraced me while her dog pulled on his leash.

We stood there talking for a while longer. I asked about her daughter, who had struggled with some anxiety issues. She told me about her daughter's counseling and the medication she was on for anxiety. I told her about Finn's horrible experience with medication and asked her if her daughter had the same difficult time. She said she didn't.

"Maybe the next prescription won't be so tough for her," I said while praying I was right. "I know they all work differently in the brain."

"They really do. Don't give up. There's one out there that will help. I'm sure."

We parted ways after a solid forty-five minutes of talking in the street.

I remembered a time when I thought other people had lives that were together and less messy than mine. But the longer I live and the more I share and connect, I realize all lives are messy. Some lives I thought were so great fell apart on closer inspection once I found out that someone in the family was an addict, getting divorced, struggling with unemployment or any number of things. People are beautiful and broken, trying their best to make a good life for themselves and those they love. We all need a little more love, patience, and sometimes even a good talk in the middle of a walk through the neighborhood.

I continued on my run, and despite my urge to mark my emotional rambling as pointless, I couldn't. A random cry in the middle of the street was actually more helpful than I would have thought. Though nothing had changed, I felt a bit less fragmented.

A few pieces closer to whole.

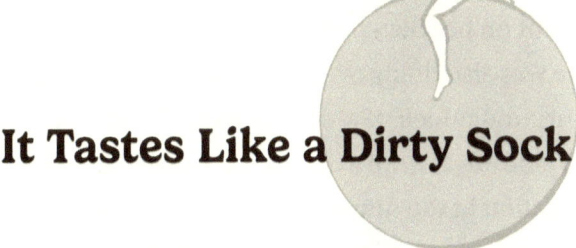

# CHAPTER 15

# It Tastes Like a Dirty Sock

It was nice to hear laughter coming from Finn's room during her new telehealth appointment. Every time she met with a new doctor; my stomach would ache. Today she was on a call with Dr. Landers, the psychiatrist Dr. Yong had referred her to, hoping to find the right medication that could calm her anxiety without sending her into panic spirals like the last one had. I heard her bounding down the stairs and took a deep breath.

"How did it go?" *She's smiling; that's a good sign.*

"Great!"

"Did you like him?"

"Yeah, he's really nice."

The dread inside my stomach uncoiled itself. "Are y'all going to be meeting again? What did he say?"

"Yes, we'll be meeting every month for a medication check in. He told me that since I'm so freaked out from the last time I was on medication; we would start really small. We discussed a lot of different drugs and the pros and cons of each and how they work. We eventually decided to try Prozac. He gave me a prescription for the liquid because he wants to start me on such a small dose that there is no tablet he could prescribe. We would have to fourth the lowest dose tablet, and he thinks it would just crumble."

I was digging the baby bird approach. There were so many things to like about Dr. Landers. He talked through everything with Finn and made her part of her own healing process instead of just writing a prescription and sending her on her way. He was working in conjunction with Finn's psychologist. But above all, Finn was using the word "we" when she referred to her appointment with him. He was making her an agent on her own path to healing.

He was also doing everything he could to ensure he didn't scare her off the whole idea of a prescription. I was truly afraid that one more scary side effect from a drug would have Finn refusing to ever consider medication in the future.

Our pharmacy didn't keep liquid Prozac in stock and had to special order it. Even after we finally got it, Finn waited several days. Her hesitancy was a testament to just how bad the side effects had been last time. There were times of, "Well, I was going to take my first dose tonight, but I've got to get up early, and it might keep me awake." "Well, maybe I should wait until the end of the semester." But eventually she started taking it.

She used a syringe to squirt it into her mouth and then stood at the kitchen counter, gagging. "Oh, God! This is terrible!"

"I'm sorry. Eventually you'll be able to take it as a pill. So, that's something to look forward to."

The gagging continued. "It tastes like dirty socks smell."

"Maybe chase it with apple juice to kill the taste."

For several weeks, she took the low dosage with no ill effects. I watched her for signs of trouble as before. She said she felt fine.

She met with the doctor again at the end of four weeks. He asked how she was tolerating the medication, and they decided that she should increase the dosage.

Once more, she did well, and they increased it again with no issues. She was finally up to the minimum dosage that could be taken in pill form, but Dr. Landers didn't want to switch to the pill at that point, as he wanted her to be able to take portions in between the two smallest pill dosages, and liquid was the easiest way to step it up slowly and carefully.

I was beyond grateful that he took her concerns and fears about the medication seriously and respected how she felt instead of just hand-ing her a prescription that she was too scared to take and throw up his hands when she reported that the side effects were terrifying her.

Although there were more instances of OCD breakdowns, her general mood seemed to improve. There was still far to go. We would learn just how far in the months to come.

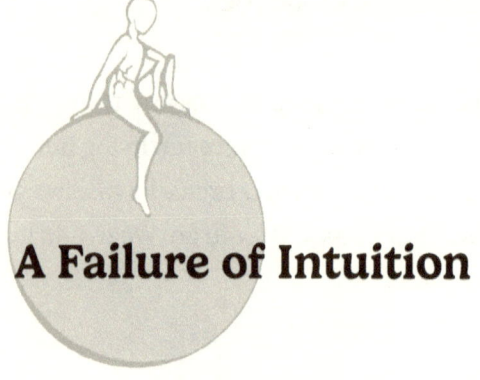

# CHAPTER 16

# A Failure of Intuition

I'd heard friends talk about how foreign taking care of children seemed to them. They joked about having no idea how to change a diaper or not knowing what in the world they would do if their child had a meltdown. I never felt this way, even before having kids. I always felt it would be innate, and it was. If one of them was upset, I knew it before they started crying. I knew if they were about to wake up before they even stirred. I would look at one of them and think *she has a fever* before I even touched her forehead, and she did. My intuition simply did not fail me, but over the last few years, I'd felt as if the universe had noticed me getting too comfortable and placed a blindfold around my third eye, sent me back into the parenting arena, and said, "you'll thank me later," or "this is for your own good," or some other bullshit that we only appreciate in hindsight.

But the past the past few years had turned everything I thought I'd known upside down. When Finn was a little girl and seemed upset, I would just talk to her, and we could work almost anything out until the OCD came along. Until then, it felt like my love was magic.

Then when I had Brea, words rarely helped at all. Her expressive receptive language disorder made it hard for her to tell me how she was feeling, and I could talk all day, but she seemed to only under-stand a portion of any given thing I said. I went from being a confident, competent mom to suddenly feeling adrift and fragmented. I was dealing with two different issues with my children, applying the same love and understanding that had worked in the past and falling further and further behind.

Don't get comfortable. The universe is watching.

At any rate, I've come to understand that being a good mom often means understanding when it is time to employ outside help. Living is a process of growing and evolving. Just when we think we have it all figured out we discover we don't, and that's okay.

Along the way I've met some of the loveliest, most patient speech therapists that have helped Brea learn to communicate and specialists to help her deal with the frustration of it all. God bless every one of them for their efforts.

And I can never be thankful enough for the mental health professionals that have helped Finn get her life back.

Perhaps my intuition didn't fail after all. Maybe intuition is just as much about knowing when it's time to go get help as it is knowing when it's time for the right words, a hug, or a rest.

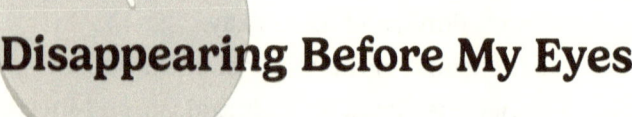

# CHAPTER 17

# Disappearing Before My Eyes

Finn sat on the couch with her head down, phone in hand, giggling as she thumbed through one screen after the other. A pause, then more giggling. The sound of her laughter was a balm to my ears and heart. Weeks had gone by with no ill side effects from her medication. The Prozac and therapy seemed to be working.

However, there were times when I felt as if I was losing her to her devices. I knew I was not the only parent to feel this way. And there was a great hesitancy on my part to give her a lecture about the amount of time she spent on them, not only because she was nineteen now, but also because I knew that her phone was a lifeline when her mind was a torment. Her thumb could race from one funny Tik Tok post to the next, and her brain didn't have time to get bogged down in the obsessive thoughts.

Brea was no exception when it came to disappearing into electronic devices. She didn't show any signs of OCD, but her speech disorder made it easier to escape into make believe than to have to talk to us when words were frustrating for her. And truthfully, I had so much to do that, let's be honest, it was easy to let them spend lots of time playing games. It could get out of hand, though, such that when I did try to talk to them, I got grunts and nods instead of conversation. The problem was that this wouldn't help Brea's communication, nor would it help Finn deal with reality.

I was forever grateful that Sean got Finn in the habit of not looking at her phone during dinnertime. To this day, it is a good time to talk to her, and those conversations often extended past the meal.

"George, I think I understand you better now," Finn said as he washed the dishes.

"Oh yeah, why's that?"

"I found this quiz that tells you what your love language is. I think your love language is acts of service. I used to worry that you would get resentful because you do so much around here, but now I think that it's just how your love expresses itself."

She was referring to a quiz based on Gary Chapman's *The Five Love Languages: How to Express Heartfelt Commitment to Your Mate.*

"It is. I love doing things for you guys."

I asked, "Did you take the quiz? What is your language?"

"I don't know. Let me see."

She worked her way through the quiz and found that her language was touch followed by quality time.

This made sense to me, as the first thing she would say if someone looked upset was, "Do you need a hug?" I had often felt that this question was based partly on the fact that she was actually the one who needed a hug.

"That's interesting," George said. "I would've guessed affirmation or something like that."

"No, and honestly, when I walk up behind mom to put my chin on her head as a joke about how tall I am, it's often because I want to be close to someone."

That was something I didn't know. I just figured it was part of her silly streak and thought it was funny that she had a tiny mama. Or, perhaps, it was scary for her to ask for a hug and approaching me in a jokey way was easier. I said, "I didn't know that! I can give you a hug anytime you like."

"Well, I didn't want to bother you."

"It never bothers me to get hugs from you."

I took the quiz next and learned that my love language was affirmation and quality time, with touch being last. I realized if I'd taken the quiz during my marriage to Sean, touch would have likely been at the top of the list since we had simply been roommates for so long. But my needs had changed and, ironically, now that I could have touch from my romantic partner, I was often stressed and the last thing I wanted was touch. Of course, a hug from a child was a whole other thing entirely, and I loved that.

George took the quiz next and discovered that his primary love language was touch, followed by acts of service. I wasn't at all surprised. He was constantly doing something for us like cleaning up, going to the grocery store, or buying me little gifts. And he would accept hugs a hundred times a day if I would give them. I think he might stand there all day long getting a hug. It did make me a little sad to hear this, as I realized that the more stressed I got, the less I wanted to be touched. I made a mental note to set aside more time and energy for hugs and kisses. He deserved them.

I watched Brea sitting on the couch playing on her computer and wondered what her love language would be. Like me, she wasn't a big hugger. She didn't really like talking either. But I realized she did give compliments and encouragement, and lately, she enjoyed telling stories—which were monologues instead of conversations. Still, these might be considered a form of spending quality time together.

She would tell grand adventure stories. George and I both noticed that she had trouble telling us what had happened during her school day. Perhaps the Mixed Expressive Receptive Language Disorder (MERLD) made it difficult to describe activities and find the right words for things that required precision and accuracy but not for stories that were made up, and she spun some epic tales.

She could tell us fiction stories that had dramatic twists and turns, original characters, and colorful worlds. She would ask me to tell stories as well but corrected me often when my imaginings didn't match hers, and then she would take over. Once such a marathon tale occurred while we were out planting blueberry bushes that spring.

"Tell me a story," Brea said in between screeching over bees that came within a ten-foot radius of her.

"One day, three little girls went on a camping trip."

"No, three teenagers."

"Okay, three teenagers went on a camping trip. They camped on a cliff above the ocean with a beautiful view. As the sun set, they sat around the campfire, and one of them said, "What is that sound?'

Sara said, 'I don't know, but it seems to be coming from the ocean.' So, they walked to the edge and saw a woman pop up out of the water and a fin disappear below the waves.

Catie said, "I see a mermaid!"

"No, no mermaids," Brea corrected.

"Okay. No mermaids. How about a sea dragon?"

"No."

"What about a—"

"Okay. I'll just tell it," Brea said.

"Lisa, Ian, and Connie fell through a portal and into an ice world, and then when they fell in, an evil water spirit lived there, and they might drown if the evil water spirit pulls them in. While they were walking, they saw this huge black cat with glowing eyes and thick fur. He is big. The same size as a lion.

Connie said, "Oh, no!" and Lisa said, "Run! But don't break the ice or the water spirit will pull us down and we might drown. But if we can run away, the evil cat might chase us . . ."

I listen intently despite being shut down from my tale of camping and mermaids.

". . . Then the polar bear growls. It's icy with lots of mountains and footprints. Connie said, 'Wait, we fell into this portal, and we went into this world, and I don't know what it's called.'"

"Wait, are they at the North Pole?"

"No, they only think they are. Ian takes a picture with his camera, and the camera tells him that they are really on Neptune with unstoppable lizards."

"Unstoppable lizards? I love it!"

"No, *blizzards.*" She enunciated the word so that my feeble ears could understand.

"Oh, my gosh! That's a good story twist, Brea. I didn't see it coming."

"I know! So, they are there a few weeks, and it turns into Neptune of darkness. I mean, Neptune of evil."

She continued her story as I broke up the ground for the blueberry plant. I realized she did want to spend time with me and sharing stories was her love language.

We all love in a different way.

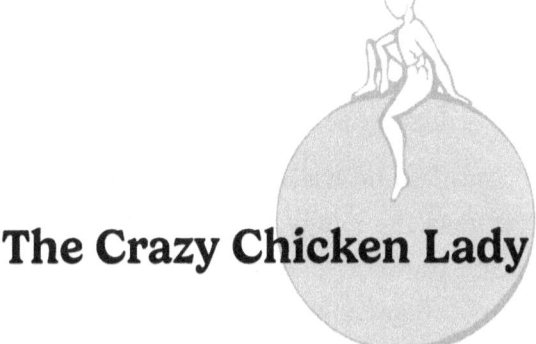

# CHAPTER 18

# The Crazy Chicken Lady

Finn had never wanted to live a typical life. She loathed living in the suburbs and craved a life that was authentically hers. There was a deep ambition to shape and live the unique life she imagined for herself, and yet she was terrified that she couldn't make it happen.

She sat at the kitchen table in her thick, wearable blanket that her dad and his girlfriend bought for her as the last hours of winter break slipped away. The blanket she wore looked like a judge's robe and when she entered the room, I called her "Your Honor." She wasn't looking forward to returning to school. It felt meaningless to her. Although she switched her major to art, she feared she wouldn't be able to find a job that was exciting. We had this conversation a lot. "I'm afraid I'm going to just end up in a job I hate, live in the suburbs, and die."

"Well, that's . . . something."

She made the same pained sound as usual. It was a mix of anguish and mirth. She knew she was providing melancholy scenarios and offering no solutions. She understood it was a tad ridiculous and fatalistic but got why it was a little amusing as well.

"I mean, what's the point? *What's* the point?"

As usual, I wanted to encourage without overwhelming, but it was a balancing act. "Your life can be as different as you want it to be. The great news is that it's all up to you. You can create the life you want."

"But there's no excitement in life."

"I think maybe you say that because you are still spending so much of your time battling OCD, and that's depressing and siphons off so much of your energy." I reminded myself that she was still on a very low dosage of Prozac, and it could take a while to build up in a person's system.

"But even without all that, how many people live the life they want?"

I got it. As Thoreau said, "The masses of men lead lives of quiet desperation." They sure do. Getting what you want out of life takes commitment and actual work. Not everyone is up to the challenge, and I was afraid to push a person already dealing with intense OCD and anxiety. Most people are simply too scared to go for what they want. "I actually know a few people that live the life they want. Believe it or not, I love my life. There are still a few things I'd like to have, and I'm working toward them, but I'm doing what I enjoy. I love being a mom. I love writing and the people in the critique groups that I'm part of. I love running. You make the life you want. You can do it. You really can. I know you can."

"Ehh." She smiled and buried her head in her hands.

"Look, when I was in my teens and even twenties and people would say this kind of thing to me, I would tell them how they didn't understand, over and over again, but in hindsight, I realize I was just scared to move forward. I was afraid that I was missing something that everyone else had. I wasn't. I had it all along, and so do you."

"But how do you *know*? How do I know my life won't be meaningless?"

"Oh, so there's OCD wrapped up in this as well."

"Yes. I don't know which part of my worries is OCD and what is a real problem anymore."

"Yeah, I can see that. Well, look at it this way, the more you stick with your therapy and untangle the OCD, the clearer the path forward will become. It's hard to know what's what when OCD has tangled itself up in your thoughts like a knotted-up necklace. You don't have to have everything figured out right now. You're only nineteen."

"But I want to know that it's worth it now."

"You can't know everything right now." *Thank you very much, OCD!*

"Look at it this way: even the confusion is a necessary part of the journey. It's the place where you grow and find out what you *really* want from life. It's okay to not have it all figured out right now."

"No, it isn't."

I felt this conversation, at first glance, seemed to be just a college student trying to figure out what direction they're going, but it was veering down the OCD highway. I was not supposed to be enabling, but with OCD you sometimes don't even know you're having a reassurance-seeking conversation until you're right in the thick of it, doing the reassuring. So, I decided that at least for today, it was unproductive. "I love you."

"I love you, too," she said in a voice that sounded painful.

Even with a prescription and fantastic therapy, OCD can linger. There have been many studies that demonstrate why this is true. In one study,[9] pairs of patients were placed in an fMRI. One patient suffered from OCD and one did not. They were then shown two faces. One face was sometimes associated with a mild shock to the wrist. The other face was not. At first, the OCD patient could associate that one face meant danger and the other didn't. However, once the faces were reversed in order of presentation, the OCD patients saw *both* faces as threatening. The neurotypical brain knew one was threatening and the other wasn't.

The researchers concluded that perhaps the OCD patient had never learned which face was safe to begin with. The non-OCD brain gave off a signal coming from the area of the brain associated with safety, the ventromedial prefrontal cortex. The OCD brain showed no signal in that area at all, not even before the images were reversed. This demonstrated that OCD patients are likely to have trouble learning and maintaining what is safe and what is not. This is why Finn knows

---

9   **See endnote 5:** Apergis-Schoute, Annemieke. (2015). "Brain Scan Reveal Why it is so Difficult to Recover From OCD-and Hint at Ways Forward." The Conversation.

she's not a murderer on a logical level, but her brain never gives her the signal that *she* is safe. If her brain never confirms this for her, she will continually circle back around to questioning it.

The results of this research bring about another issue that may need therapeutic treatment: learning. How does one *learn* what is safe instead of simply not reacting to the compulsions that are a *result* of not feeling safe? Currently, cognitive behavioral therapy is directed at the manifestation of not feeling safe: compulsions and rituals. This suggests that the root of the OCD could use more work and research. Perhaps in the future, there will be targeted therapy at training the brain to recognize what is safe, in addition to the current therapy.

The next evening, I heard George and Finn talking in the kitchen. Finn was laughing—a sound I'm always grateful to hear.

"There are plenty of places where you could have chicken or goat and still live near a progressive town that would be LGBTQ friendly. You wouldn't have to live in the city," I heard George say.

"Yeah, that would be good because I want to have a little patch of land to put a tiny house on, too."

"Let's see . . . There's Asheville, North Carolina. There's Black Mountain," George continued.

I finished up some chores while they talked, and when I walked into the room, George said, "Finn has something she wants to show you."

She showed me notes on her phone, bullet points even, and explained each one. "Okay, so I've decided that since I couldn't figure out whether I wanted to live in the country or the city, I could just get a tiny house and move into the country on a piece of land that is *near* a progressive city."

"Oh, I like it." She showed me notes about Black Mountain, North Carolina, a place she and George had discussed. "What else?"

"I figure I can get a chicken, maybe a few, or a goat. I want to still live close enough that you can come visit, of course."

"Of course! I can bring you food. George can bring you jars of his mother's spaghetti sauce recipe. This is fun. Tell me more."

"Okay, well, I can work a part-time job while I'm in college. Also, I'm going to need a cat or a dog to keep me company." She stopped and thought, scratching her head for a moment. "A dog will need me to get up early and let it out. Eh, maybe just a cat. But I could teach a cat to walk with a leash, if I get started early enough."

We'd tried putting a cat on a leash before. It seemed to believe it was being attacked and ran through the house like it was on fire, the leash dragging behind it. I was skeptical of this part of her plan but let it go.

"Vincent and I agreed that if either of us ever needed a place to live that we would let the other come live with us."

"Ah, that's so nice," George said from where he stood drying a frying pan in the kitchen.

"Yeah, I'll have to tell him all about my idea."

"You should! This is wonderful. I'm very excited about visiting you in the mountains."

"Me too!"

Later that night when I went to bed, I heard her laughing on the phone as she told Vincent all about her ideas to live in the country with chickens. Sometimes parents are like the biblical prophet with no honor in their land. It took someone like George with a fresh perspective, who isn't tied up in parental memories and prejudices, to help her see a whole new perspective. I didn't think it would change everything for her, and it didn't.

The next day she was asking what would happen if she moved to the tiny house in the country and became miserable. I started to reply but then just smiled and said, "I love you."

I didn't know if the medication was helping her see her way clear or if she was simply maturing, but at least she was beginning to imagine a life beyond the room where she paced holes in the carpet, and that was enough.

At least for today.

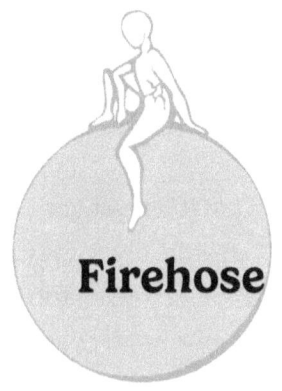

# CHAPTER 19

**Firehose**

I've heard medication for neurological issues referred to as "happy pills." But people who are suffering with mental illness would likely say, "I wish!" For Finn, and many like her, the medication is simply something to lower the anxiety so that they may be able to effectively do the Cognitive Behavioral Therapy (CBT), specifically Exposure and Response Prevention (ERP), that is so necessary for OCD sufferers. If someone with OCD can't even begin to do the work it takes to get better because of high anxiety levels, then they could remain stuck for years, and Finn had been. Far from being "happy pills," the medication simply gives the individual the opportunity to be on a level playing field, neurologically speaking, so they can making progress with their mental health.

Though Finn's overall disposition did seem steadier while on Prozac, she still had meltdowns once or twice a month. George dubbed these episodes the "firehose." Firehose was accurate because she'd go from idle chit chat to talking really fast about what was bothering her and crying to the point of almost hyperventilating.

These firehose moments seemed to happen whenever I got too comfortable believing Finn was making real progress on her medication. They generally took place in the evening. It would start with a concern about not getting her schoolwork done in time, having to take a dead-end job when she gets out of college and then die old and miserable, or never being able to find a partner to love. While these are legitimate concerns that any college student might have, they would spiral into a full-on episode with OCD firmly mixed in with the fear. It would often be difficult to dissect the legitimate concerns from the

OCD tendencies. OCD deals in absolutes—that's always an OCD red flag.

"What if I never get a girlfriend?"

"You will."

"What if I find a girlfriend and say the wrong thing?"

"At some point everyone says the wrong thing. If you really like each other then you two will talk about it, and it will be fine."

"Maybe I don't want to find someone because if I screw it up it will hurt so bad that it would be better to just never meet someone, then I won't have to worry about screwing it up."

"You can't live like that. It's self-induced isolation. Everybody messes up at some point. It will be okay."

"It's exhausting to have to always worry about saying the right thing. Maybe it's easier to be alone, but I don't want to be alone."

"Then don't be. That's up to you."

"I'm scared I'm always going to be alone."

She would cry on the couch for another hour or so. I would hug and console. Of course, as a mom I also tried to reassure, but I had to be careful about that. General pep talks could cross the line into enabling the OCD. It was exhausting for us both.

"I'm going to have to get Brea to sleep soon, but we can talk some more. We can even talk tomorrow if you like."

"I'm afraid there won't be another chance. We'll go on about our day and won't get back to it."

"I'm not always sure when you're in the mood to talk. Please just come get me when you need to talk. I'm always here for you."

"But we won't."

"Of course, we will. Just come get me."

"I'll get busy. You'll get busy, and it won't happen."

"Then make it happen. Just tell me."

She burst into tears again and we talked some more. These talks often devolved into the same questions and answers on a loop, and I knew that this is part OCD and part of growing up and waiting for the brain to finish developing.

At some point, I had to leave to go tuck Brea into bed. On the one hand, I worried that Finn would feel like I was abandoning her for Brea just as she thought I did when she was younger and wanting my attention, but baby Brea would start crying. On the other hand, during these firehose meltdowns I worried that I was enabling her anyway, and my reassurance became a crutch. Perhaps having a solid end time to these conversations was a good thing. It was impossible to know. I always felt just a little torn.

I gave Finn a big hug before heading upstairs. When I came back downstairs, she didn't seem to want to talk anymore.

The next day, my fiancé and I were waiting in line to pick up my youngest from school. Ahead of us was a long line of cars snaking through the parking lot. Inside the cars sat parents staring at phones, listening to the radio, or maybe just enjoying a moment away from their home office and endless Zoom meetings that had become the normal way of doing things during the pandemic.

George asked, "Do you notice that Finn is fine the next day after one of those 'firehose' episodes?"

"Yeah, when I was her age, I would do that and move on. What else can someone do?"

"So, you think those feelings are always there, and they just build up until they burst?"

"Well, yeah." I was fascinated that this seemed so foreign to him, and I wonder if it is a gender thing. I thought back to my days in high school where girls would be crying in bathrooms, making themselves late for class while they had a meltdown as their friends tried to help or joined them in the emotional fray. "I think these are fears she always has, and then the worry over them gets to be too much, and the firehose turns on. Do you think it all gets out and then she should be fine and move on?"

"Well, yeah, I guess I would, but I'm sunny Jim," he said.

I laughed. "You're not normal."

"Nope. Do you ever worry about the effect it has on Brea? You know, she sees these meltdowns and maybe she worries that she's going to be that way when she gets to be a teenager?"

"That's a good point, but she just really seems unaffected by it. I think she might be too absorbed in her own world to worry about it."

"True. She doesn't seem bothered by it."

I contemplated this as she got in the car. I remembered the night she asked a sobbing Finn if a teddy bear would help her feel better.

Should I be doing more to protect her from her sister's meltdowns? Kids across the world had big sisters or brothers having teenage angst. Did other parents rush the older children into another room the moment they got upset? Was that even healthy? Did it make the emotions seem like something dangerous or wrong through the eyes of the younger sibling? Frustration and grief are part of life. Honestly, I was not sure.

Just as Finn must deal with the uncertainty for her OCD to ever get better, so parents have to deal with the uncertainty of never quite knowing if what we are doing is the very best thing for our children.

Finn was right. Uncertainty sucked.

CHAPTER 20

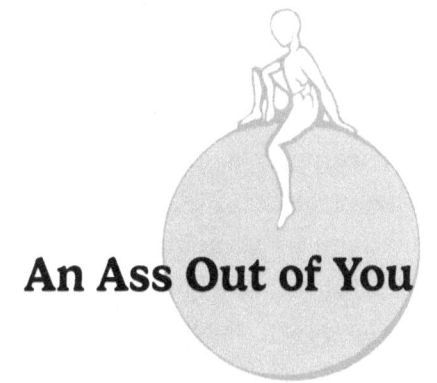

# An Ass Out of You

As bad as Harm OCD can torment, there were other intrusive thoughts that came really close to being an equal menace.

One night, Finn sat on the couch after Brea had gone to bed and turned on the proverbial firehose. "My room was the one place where I could feel calm. Now I can't even relax in there."

"Why?"

"Because I'm afraid I'm being watched. I mean, I know I'm not being watched, logically. But I wonder if somehow someone from one of my posters can see me. I wonder if maybe someone is looking through a crack in the blinds. I have to sit at a certain spot in my room that is away from anything that I feel like may watch me. I don't *believe* anyone is watching me. It's like the Harm OCD. Logically, I don't believe that I'm a murderer. You know? It's just that I have a fear that in some weird way it might be possible."

My mind went back again to the studies cited in *Brain Lock*[10] about the door being left open to any illogical thought. Finn and even I, now and then, hang a sign somewhere in our brain, "All thoughts welcome. No thought too weird or bizarre." I think there might even be an evil clown dancing around below it.

As I listened to her explaining where she had to sit in her room in order to be safe from the eyes that she knows aren't really watching her, I realized that if someone didn't understand OCD, they might

10    **See endnote 1:** Schwartz, Jeffrey, and Beyette, Beverly. (2016). *Brain Lock: Free Yourself from Obsessive-Compulsive Behavior: A Four-Step Self-Treatment Method to Change Your Brain Chemistry.* New York: Harper Perennial, page 50

have assumed that this being-watched phobia is some sort of paranoid schizophrenia. Just like some people wrongly assume that OCD is someone that's obsessed with neatness.

But there are assumptions from within as well. Even those who've had OCD and should have no assumptions, still make them. I assumed when she went to the first psychiatrist's office that they would be able to help her, but that wasn't the reality.

I assumed that when she went to that first counselor, she would crack open the vault to her mind and tell them what she needed in order to be well again. It wasn't that easy. What little they had taught her about OCD at school left her believing that there was no way she had it. We often assume any data is good, but with conflicting data, we end up being wrong more often than not. Therefore, she didn't bother getting into it. And perhaps, she was picking up on my fear of her talking about it. There are layers of assumption and misunderstanding that stand in the way of recovering.

I also made assumptions about how she would handle OCD. When my symptoms were at their peak, I didn't deal with the moral and religious aspects of it as much. I didn't worry as much about what people thought. Finn worries more about how every single move she makes affects others.

We've had the same conversations many times.

"I get tired of feeling like I always have to make sure everyone is okay. I'm sick of it. I don't know if they're angry or not. So, I'm always trying to make sure other people aren't angry at me. But if I make them happy, then I can't be happy."

"Why not?"

"Because if I'm trying to make someone happy, it means that I'm worried they're mad at me, which means I'm stressed out. But then at least if they aren't mad at me, then I look great for being nice, but the motivation is selfish because I just want everyone to be happy with me. On the other hand, if they're doing something for *me,* then they must be upset and trying to placate me."

"That must be exhausting for you." I feel sad that almost any moment she isn't in her room, pacing, listening to music, or playing video games, is emotionally draining for her.

"It is exhausting. If I'm happy, then other people aren't happy because I'm not doing anything for them. It's like we can't all be happy at the same time."

"Oh, my God, Finn. That's . . ."

"I know, right?! They say, 'if it ain't broke don't fix it,' but I can't tell if it's broke so I'm going to fix it anyway."

I thought back to the study with the faces and how the person with OCD couldn't tell which face was safe and which one was associated with the shock. "I'm happy with you when you aren't doing anything for me. I'm just glad to be with you."

"You're my mom."

"Yes, but not everyone is selfish. You don't have to constantly monitor what people are thinking."

"Yes, I do. I want to be loved, but I can't because I'm making them sad. I'm creating a burden for them. Because they are trying to make me happy because I've been upset in some way."

"Everybody wins but you."

"Right. What if you think this OCD stuff is your fault?" she asks me.

"Why would I think that?"

"Because it runs in your family."

"Well, sure, but I don't think like that. It's just genetics."

"But what if you do?"

"I don't."

"But what if you do?"

"I don't. But look, you might get a foot tumor from your dad's side of the family, and that wouldn't be his fault either. Who cares? It's just genetics. This is a lot of power to assign to yourself."

Finn laughed. "Yeah, Dr. Yong said to me, 'Wow! How does it feel to have all that God like power?'"

"Exactly. If you were talking to someone else about this stuff, and they thought they were responsible for some genetic thing they had no control over, how would you respond?"

"I would be compassionate to them and say it doesn't matter, because it doesn't."

"But you can't extend that same sort of mercy to yourself?"

"No. You might as well sell me to a witch in the woods."

"Why?"

"Because she will ask for your firstborn child as currency."

Finn has a remarkable gift for being able to find humor in some really horrible emotional caves. I'm convinced it's been given to her by God in anticipation of all the turmoil she deals with. So why not just hold the humor and the OCD as well? I don't know, but I believe how we all handle it matters, and someday we will understand.

I wonder if I didn't go through this type of OCD because I understood early on that there were some people that I simply could not make happy no matter how hard I tried. My stepmother was one of them. When she was in the middle of a rage, there was nothing anyone could say to make her happy. Eventually, I learned to just stop trying. From that time forward, I knew that some people insist on misery and will take you with them if you allow it. But here I am, even as someone who has suffered through OCD, trying to apply logic to it. I should know by now, there is no rationale with this disorder. Or perhaps, my OCD is a house cat and Finn's is a tiger. One might assume ours would be roughly the same, but it isn't.

There are also some who believe that someone who does ERP won't need meds. While this may be true for an uncle, cousin, or next-door neighbor, this might not be true for yourself or a loved one. Treatment can vary based on the individual and how many other factors are involved. Some people have other neurological issues going on at the same time.

I also assumed there were battles I would have to continually fight.

One must be very careful about this. If we always have our sword up, we might challenge the wrong person. I suspected Dr Landers, Finn's new psychiatrist who regulates her meds, would be one more battle I might need to fight, but it turned out great. We get so used to having to fight that we forget what it is like to live in peace.

It's human to make assumptions because we want to make the future less scary.

Perhaps one of the worst assumptions one could make would be assuming that OCD can be cured. It can't. But the symptoms can be managed and lessened to the point that we feel the tendency, just below the surface, like I do, but know better than to give it an inch. I never assume it couldn't still seize power. Every time I feel that compulsion to check the lock just one more time, to read that sentence again to ensure I don't get cancer, or when I have a random violent thought, I know to keep my thoughts "loose." "Don't grab," I say to myself—a metaphor I use when I feel the urgency to assure myself with ritual or thought.

I know, with certainty, that every time I grab, something grabs back.

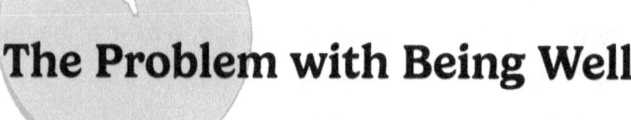

# CHAPTER 21

# The Problem with Being Well

After George moved into the house, there was definitely a learning curve. He didn't have any kids and suddenly, all the time that was focused solely on us when we were dating, was now divided. Even when we were alone together, sometimes my mind would be on my kids. Even though he loves Finn and Brea and gets along well with them, the burden of their wellbeing will never weigh as heavily on his shoulders and mind as it does on mine.

We have a friend with a lovely cabin in the North Georgia mountains who invited us to use it for the weekend. When I'm away from my kids for that long, I still initially have the feeling that I should be doing something for them. I continue to feel anxious for a few hours until it settles in that no one is going to ask me for anything.

We sat on the porch and enjoyed the view of the mountains through the rustling orange, red, and yellow leaves still clinging to the branches. We had time to write, talk, and go out to dinner at a local restaurant while the kids spent time with their dad and his girlfriend. George and I talked over drinks while we waited for our entrees to arrive.

"So, when do you think you'll be able to get Brea to sleep by herself?"

I took a drink of my coconut cocktail to try to buy some time for myself. Brea had slept next to me when she was a baby and nursing. Like my first daughter, I had trouble getting her back into her bed after waking up to nurse. Unlike when Finn was born, though, I gave up trying to get her back into bed and just let her sleep next to me. After losing two babies before her, I worried something would happen to her during the night. I would later learn that this was not uncommon for moms who have lost babies. Not only that, but there is also an interesting thing that happens when you have children later in life: you're so damn tired, you don't worry about the same things you did with your first child.

I also have to admit that Brea's presence in our bed kept Sean and I from having to deal with awkward relationship issues. The fact that those issues deepened as the years went on resulted in Brea being eight years old and still sleeping beside me.

When George moved in, I thought I could get Brea to sleep in her own room, and she did—but she cried until I slept up there with her. I knew she was having a difficult time with all the changes going on, so I thought I would just sleep up there with her for a little while. However, she told me she didn't like George for pushing her out of my bedroom, and I worried that me leaving her upstairs and going downstairs to sleep next to George would give her yet another reason to resent him.

I was struggling to keep everyone happy. In the meantime, my back was hurting from sharing a twin bed with an eight-year-old who sprawled like her father and left me little room to get comfortable.

George was still waiting for my answer. I told him, "I know that when I launch into trying to get her to sleep alone it's going to be night after night of her crying herself to sleep. That just feels like more stress than I can handle right now. Besides, I have to admit that sleeping up there has given *me* some adjustment time as well. But I know this must be tough on you."

"Well, I have to admit, I didn't move in with you just so I could be ignored."

"That's valid, and I don't want you to be miserable. But I'm trying to make you, Brea, and Finn happy, and what I want doesn't matter." To my surprise I found myself getting angry.

"Yes, it does. I want you to be happy. What you need matters."

"No, it doesn't, and you know it!" I struggled to avoid crying.

"Yes, it does. So, what I hear is that you need more space from me."

He'd told me several times since we got together that he would be happy if he could be with me around the clock, that he would never tire of being with me. This made me feel bad because I'm the type of person who needs alone time. But anytime we stifle our own needs, we end up in resentful relationships. I knew I had to be honest about my needs.

"I think so. Yes. I don't want you to go anywhere. I love you, and I want you with me. It's just a lot of pressure to go from having just kids that wanted my affection and just being able to focus on them, to suddenly having someone who wants my attention like you do."

It was hard to relax and give him my undivided attention. He is kind, attentive, giving everything that I've always wanted, and yet, I found it hard to be happy.

This is the relationship I always hoped for. One where my partner and I shared interests and felt passionate about the same things. He does all the things that would have been on my wish list. Yet, when I go out for a jog, where I do my best thinking, I ask myself, am I just ungrateful? Why can't I just be happy?

I'm not the only one with this type of problem.

Finn told me she was afraid that once she got the OCD under control, there would be nothing that defined her. "I don't want to be one of those spoiled, entitled people that have everything so easy."

"You won't. You will be forever changed by this experience. Trust me, when this is under control, there will be something else, perhaps not as intense, but there will still be life. There will still be challenges."

"I know. At some point, I should be happy to be better.

"I get it, but now you can be defined by something positive instead of something tormenting."

"Yeah," she said, but still appears deep in thought. These questions of identity are something we have to work out on our own. No one can tell us who we are, how we define ourselves, or what makes us happy.

All these things played through my head as I ran. When I was married to Sean, I was lonely, but I didn't have to give anything either. We were roommates. We expected little out of each other because we both knew the other didn't have it to give. But now, I have someone who loves me so much that he wants my time, my attention, and frankly, it was exhausting.

*Just be happy* for God's sake. But it wasn't that easy. And maybe it wasn't supposed to be. Much like Sisyphus, we all have a rock to push up a hill. That is neither good nor bad. It's just life. I would even argue we need that rock. We need to wake up every day and deal with it and that's okay. A state of permanent bliss is no bliss at all but a lie.

Pushing that rock up the hill forces us to cultivate joy inside, no matter what the outside brings.

One early morning after we dropped Brea at school, I was eating my cereal without making eye contact. I enjoy getting up early, but I do not want to talk or touch or make decisions. George always wakes up fully refreshed and energized. That morning, he was smiling and talkative. He sighed, and I didn't know what it meant. He seemed happy. Insufferably happy.

"Why do you do that?"

"What?"

"The sighing."

"Oh, because I'm happy to see you and . . ." he thinks for a moment ". . . content."

"But my hair is frizzy, and I'm grouchy. How can you be happy?"

"I just am because I love you, and we're together."

"But I'm a real pain in the ass in the morning."

"No, you're not."

"Yes, I am. Don't lie."

He smiles. "I know, but you're that way to everyone in the morning, not just me."

I feel bad about being so awful in the morning, but I always feel tired, more tired than when I go to bed at night. Everything seems overwhelming when I first wake up. Yet George sat there contentedly, sighing. He's a good man. An oddly cheerful man.

But I know that I have to learn to exist in this relationship that gives

166 ⊙ KIM CONREY with FINN CONREY

me so much. I have to learn to shift out of solo survival mode, and Finn will have to do the same when she gets what she wants: when the OCD is no longer front and center, when she's able to enjoy a moment without OCD clawing at the door.

She has been getting those moments more and more. I've heard her laughing on a regular basis. There have been far fewer meltdowns. Far less "firehose" moments.

The kids were getting older and working through their problems, as all kids have to, OCD or not. Although it seemed like a lot, it wouldn't always.

But there was a problem with being well. When we get there, it won't look like what we expected.

And that's okay.

That is life.

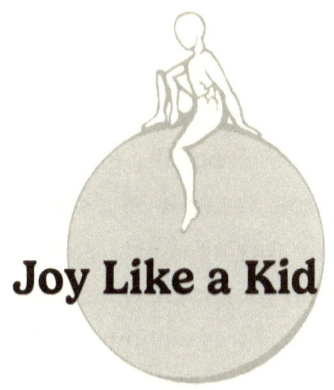

# CHAPTER 22

# Joy Like a Kid

With all the things Finn has put off or forgotten, she has always taken her Prozac. She wanted to get better, and it was working.

She sat in the kitchen talking to me as I chopped vegetables for dinner. "When I was walking to school yesterday, I noticed the texture of the moss growing along the sidewalk. When I was a kid, I used to notice things like that, and it made me happy."

I felt such joy over that revelation. This was bigger than anyone could know. The joy had been completely sapped from Finn's life for so many years. "When you were a kid, I remember you stopping on the way into the house and running your fingers across the wood grain on the siding. You took the time to really look at it. I think some of the things we notice and enjoy when we are younger are so much closer to who we really are inside and what we truly want. Also, as an artist, it makes sense that you have a love of texture."

"Yeah. I told Dr. Yong about it, and she said the medication is working. Now I'm able to be in the moment."

"Exactly. It helped free up your brain enough to get out of your head and enjoy your life more. Still no side effects?"

"No. I don't think so."

I whispered a prayer of thanks.

### Finn says:

When I first went on Prozac, I was really worried that it was going to be like my last attempt at the anti-anxiety meds. The dosage of the previous drug, Lexapro, had been too high, and it quickly made everything worse. But this time, my new psychiatrist took this information and not only started me on something different but also gave me the option to take it in a liquid form so I could start it on a small and barely noticeable dose and move my way up slowly, so my body could get used to it more easily. This took more time, but after the horrible experience I had last time, I was willing to move slowly.

I didn't realize how much it had changed my mood and perception of life until I was on it for a while. Eventually, I realized I was much calmer and more willing to forgive myself when I made mistakes. Some of my mental health problems and barriers to recovery stemmed from my self-esteem issues. I held other people in higher regard than myself, and I was unwilling to let things go if I made a mistake, but with a combination of therapy and meds, I noticed I was able to start letting some of the old habits go. I was feeling calmer, more in control of my life, and much happier in general.

All of this makes sense when you consider that I am taking an SSRI, which is a drug that helps one's brain to regulate serotonin properly. My brain creates the correct amount of serotonin but flushes it out too quickly. Like if I ate a full course meal but then immediately threw it back up. You don't get any nutrients from that and if you do, it is a small amount. In the brain, this translates to feeling nervous far more easily, and it can become hard to feel positive emotions. I felt like I was walking around in a haze all the time and really nervous because I couldn't see clearly, and it felt like I didn't know how to feel better. It all happened so gradually I didn't realize how bad it was.

Similarly, once I started taking Prozac, I didn't realize I was getting better. Because the dose was so low, and my doctor and I raised it so slowly I didn't see any big changes. It wasn't until someone asked me how I felt that I realized I was actually much calmer and less nervous. The fact that I was calmer also let me experience more happiness than I had before, since I wasn't always so stressed.

After that, I asked other people around me if I seemed any different, and they all said I was much happier and calmer. Granted this was during the pandemic, and I only had like three people to ask, but it still counts. After that, as my dose went up, I paid more attention to how I was feeling and my actions. Things really changed. Besides being much calmer, I was also much more patient, and I could be in the moment, which was another problem I was having. I had a hard time being present due to always being worried about something, and while I am still sometimes not present, I am much more than before. I can appreciate the textures of my blankets and the sounds that different things make, like sand or wind. Which may not sound like much, but I wanted to be able to experience life and truly enjoy it. It had been an experience I thought I had lost to time, because I had done those things when I was little but stopped when my OCD got bad. I also enjoy existing more. I enjoy the things I am doing while I do them.

While things have improved a lot, I still have work to do. I might need to raise my dose some more to help with some more of the therapy or I might not; time will tell. I want to be clear though, that it doesn't remove all my OCD, worry, and fear. I still have daily OCD rituals, and I still get really anxious sometimes. The point of the medicine is not to take away those things, but to make them more manageable. Before, the fear when I was doing OCD therapy seemed like it dragged me down and it kept me from making progress during my therapy sessions. I was just stagnant, trying to get better but not going anywhere. And, believe me, I tried. After the Lexapro situation, I didn't want to use medication unless there was no other option, and I only took meds again because after several months of work that was barely progressing at all, my therapist suggested I start it in order to make more progress and not be so agonizingly distressed whenever I did my ERP practice.

Some distress is fine. In fact, the exercise is about getting over stress and realizing it is okay, but when it is so bad that there is no room in your mind for effective therapy, they suggest medication to help get the ball rolling. But you still have to do the practice and go through the stress that it brings.

The next evening, she was sitting on the couch, looked up from her phone, and said, "The other evening I was in my room playing one of my games and just enjoying what I was doing, and I thought, *Wait a minute. I'm happy.* I was spontaneously happy just to be where I was. Like when I was a kid. You know? I thought that was a thing of the past, and no one felt happy again when they were adults. At least, not like that."

"Oh, my gosh! I'm so happy to hear you say that. That's wonderful!"

People can have various reactions to antidepressants, and some argue that it destroys personality. I would counter that in Finn's case Prozac didn't cover her personality, it *recovered* it and brought it out of hiding. Her personality could emerge from the bunker where it had been huddled all these years while she spent her mental energy just trying to fight this beast.

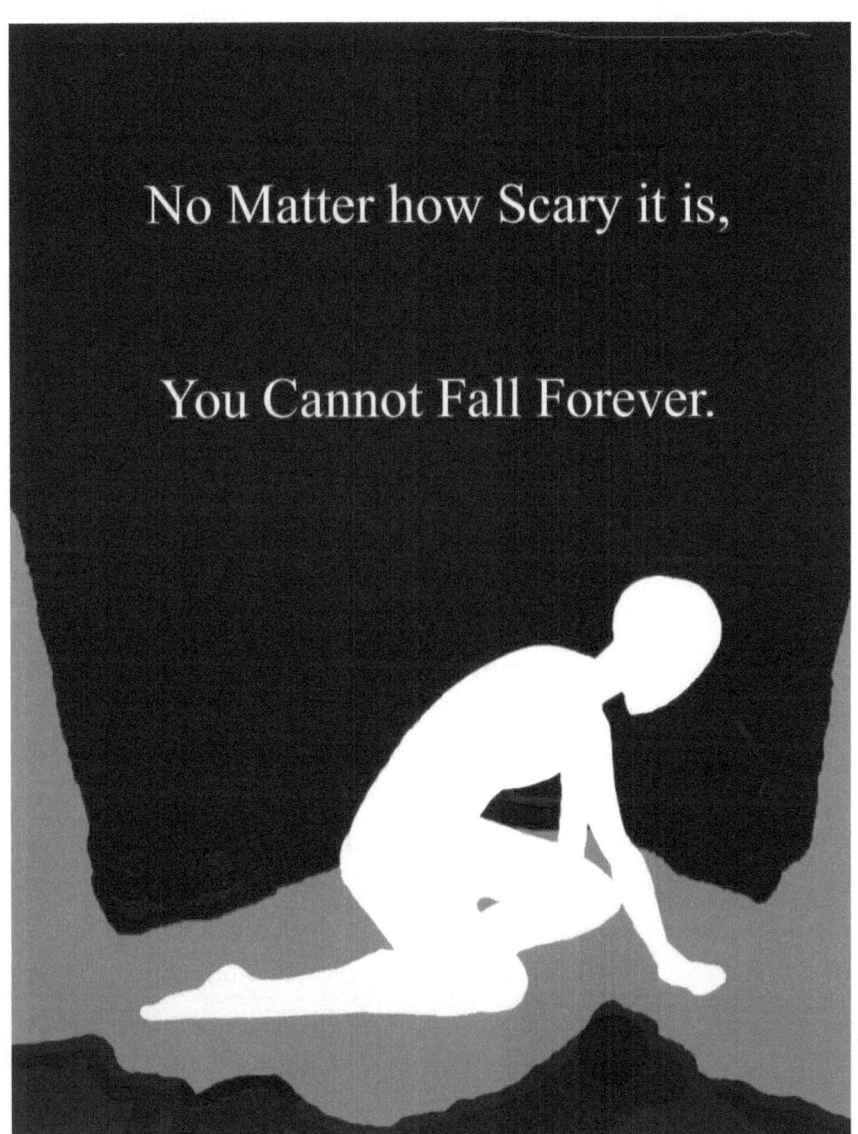

No Matter how Scary it is,

You Cannot Fall Forever.

**Illustration by Finn Conrey**

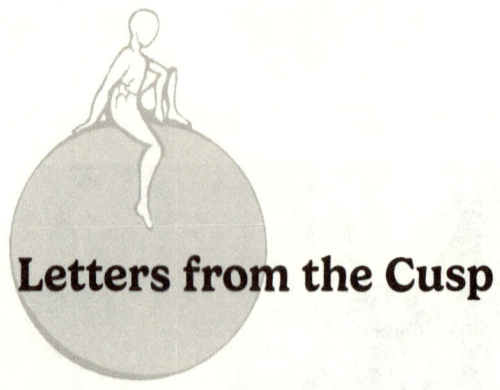

# CHAPTER 23

# Letters from the Cusp

Finn was now at the lower end of Prozac dosage for the standard treatment of OCD, which is 40 to 80 mg/day. She was still tolerating it well, with no side effects. We can attribute much of this to her psychiatrist starting her off at such a small dosage. They began at 4 mg. The patience on the part of Dr. Landers and Dr. Yong not to push for a standard dose right off is something I will always be grateful for. The predominating advice is usually to tolerate the symptoms for two weeks until your brain gets used to it. This was what happened with the Lexapro, and it almost scared her off medication for life, and the meds have been a godsend. It allowed her to move forward with the treatment that she so desperately needed.

As spring came around, we got the urge to grill. The smell of hardwood charcoal and hamburgers filled the backyard. We brought out potato salad and iced tea and enjoyed the mild weather before the sweltering Atlanta humidity and mosquitos made eating outside miserable. After we were finished with lunch, George gathered an armful of dishes and went inside. He always pointed out that Finn and I had our best talks after a meal, so he would quietly do the dishes so we could slip into conversation. Brea was in school, and Finn and I were left outside on a beautiful day with precious time to talk.

"Do you ever get the idea that something is wrong with me other than the OCD?"

*Oh, dear God, no.* "No, I don't think so." Whether she thought something was wrong or there really was, didn't matter, the emotional turmoil could be just as exhausting for her.

"Well, you were telling me about the study with the faces and how some people with OCD couldn't read emotion on faces well, you know like people with autism sometimes can't. Maybe I have a touch of autism as well."

"Well, they certainly can be comorbid, but the study wasn't suggesting that. They were specifically looking at people with OCD, and after being given an SSRI [selective serotonin reuptake inhibitor] they didn't have that problem."[11]

"Yeah. It's just that I don't want to point anyone in the wrong direction while we're writing about this if they might have autism or something."

"That's why we stress the need for anyone struggling with mental health to see a professional. Then that professional will decide what they do or don't have. This isn't an attempt to tell people what they have, but to share our story. No one should try and diagnose themselves based on a book, and you can't control it if they do. All we can do is stress the need for appropriate, qualified mental health. Maybe you are applying your OCD to our memoir now."

"How? I just don't want people to go in the wrong direction."

"Yeah, I understand that, but that's why they need to seek professional help. We're just telling a story and sharing what we have discovered, that's it. We've already stressed the need for appropriate professional help."

"Yeah."

For the rest of the day, I thought about what she had said. Even as someone is stabilizing with OCD, there can be a thousand ways that it will slip into daily life, making it hard to separate what are logical, justified concerns and what is OCD.

It occurred to me that the autism assumption could lead back around to her idea that once the OCD is under control, she will have nothing that sets her identity apart and she might appear as one more

---

11   **See endnote 6:** Jansen, M., Overgaauw, S. & De Bruijn, E. (2020). Social Cognition and Obsessive-Compulsive Disorder: A Review of Subdomains of Social Functioning.

suburbanite girl with no worries. That will never be the case though—and I'd argue there's no such thing as a worry-free existence anyway, no matter who you are or where you live. It could never be the scenario with Finn, anyway. If she wasn't struggling with being different because she's queer, then she will always have OCD. Then again, even though I'm her mom, I'm not in her head. Some people do have autism and OCD as well. It isn't that unusual, and everything would be fine if she did. I have a couple of autistic family members. They're just fine as they are. They aren't problems that need to be fixed either.

But ultimately, I can't help but wonder why anyone would want to continue defining themselves by their struggle. I will always have OCD, but I'm a writer, a runner, a mom. Why can't she be Finn the artist? Or Finn the LGBTQ lobbyist or something? Are those things scarier because she believes it takes something she doesn't have? I know she has everything she needs to be an artist, an advocate, a statue-esq, badass, queer world changer.

But perhaps defining oneself by any of those positive things wakes the OCD dragon as well. Once again, the Steinbeck quote ran through my head. *Now that you don't have to be perfect, you can be good.* Maybe she believed that if she endeavored to begin anything other than illness, she would have to be perfect at it. The OCD would demand it, and it would be so exhausting that she wouldn't be able to handle it. I'm not sure.

And that's the hard part for me. She was nineteen, and I couldn't live her life for her or tell her what she should be doing. She would have to find her own way. Pushing too hard would only lead to resentment. Ultimately, our journey is our own. That's both good and bad news, and how we perceive that depends on how strong we are feeling at any given time.

At the beginning of a journey as difficult as a child with severe OCD, we picture a day when things are better, brighter, but here at the cusp of better and brighter, there are still hurdles. Big ones. Like the need to walk into the light and claim it as her own.

I often wonder if people with Harm OCD spend so much time not only defining themselves by the worst thing they've done but the worst thing they've *thought* they might do, that defining themselves by something positive seems downright risky. The OCD demands that they be hypervigilant, always assuming the worst so that they can prevent it. The moment they start to lighten up, loosen their grip, the OCD attempts to drag them back into the dark. OCD is a master tangler. It tangles up in thought when the disorder is at its worst and then when they start to get their symptoms under control it clings to their identity like a habit that no longer serves.

If you ask me who someone is, my first thought will be all the positive attributes about them. I believe we are defined by those things. We are defined by the God in us, whatever that ideal is from culture to culture, person to person, it is this same spark, that calls us to come up higher. That's our reality, not what we struggle with.

She's always been such a bulldog about making sure she does the right thing when she thought it kept someone else safe, that when she sees her way clear to apply that same tenacity to something positive, it will send out ripples that will affect more people than she could possibly imagine.

For now, I can't rush or pressure her. For that matter, I can't even tell her what she does or doesn't have. As well as I know her, I don't know exactly what it's like to *be* her. I'm not a doctor either. Only a mental health professional could determine if she has an autism component. It's possible. I just want to be her advocate while she continues to improve and find out what makes her authentically joyful.

Watching someone recover is a great place to be, but it can be fraught with pitfalls as we caregivers observe their potential emerging from layers of oppression. There is a temptation to push too much too soon. We've seen our loved ones shackled for so long. We want everything for them right now but must consider that our encouragement might come off as pressure, and our good intentions might backfire.

They didn't develop OCD overnight and the path forward won't always be as clear or as quick as we might want either.

Progress is to be celebrated and sometimes only seen in hindsight.

## Finn says:

When I was younger, it somehow got into my head that I was a person who could only be a certain way. I had decided that expressing how I feel unless it was a very specific emotion was incorrect. Other people were allowed to change and be different, but I was being bad or untrue to myself if I did what made me happy. I think it was also partially that way because when I was little, to be cool or strong, you had to reject feminine styles and being "girly" made you weak. But I didn't want to be super masculine either. I had to keep a certain amount of female associated traits, the most obvious being I had to keep my long hair. Everyone loved my long hair and after a while I associated it with who I was as a person, and to chop it off would be bad because everyone around me loved it. After a while I grew to hate it though. All of the other things I used to feel defined me, became a prison. If I ever strayed from what was "the right choice" then I was being "bad" and I needed to fix it. My therapist would most certainly point out the OCD "black and white thinking" here.

I resented who I was and became jealous of other people, who could live how they wanted without feeling like some tragedy or punishment would befall them if they ever messed up, and immediately feeling guilty if they changed. This eventually came to a head when I went to the library one day and saw a romance manga that had some magic mixed in, so I was interested. But according to my rigid thinking I could not like romance, and if I did it would go against everything I *should* stand for, but I wanted to read it really bad, so I became stuck just worrying about what I should do, so much so that I cried in the middle of the library, over a book that I hadn't even read. My mom came over and led me out of the library at that point, and after a short car ride, she suggested I go see a therapist. It ended up not being that helpful though because we thought it was just anxiety and we didn't get to the root of the problem.

I eventually did cut my hair to shoulder length. It just got to where I resented it so badly that I just wanted it gone. But then after a while I felt as though it wasn't enough and while I was with my latest therapist, I cut it even shorter, I even colored it, I let my sister choose the color because I knew she would pick something girly—it's pink—so I could come out of my shell even more and convince myself that feminine colors are not bad and don't make you weak or less than. And now I feel a lot happier with myself. I have even started to wear dresses and skirts in daily life and mix feminine and masculine styles.

I feel more like myself than I ever did in the past when I was forcing myself only to be one way. I also am starting to feel better about having my own opinions and ideas, because before I also had to be and act a certain way when it came to those too. I felt like if I changed, I was betraying all of the people I listened to when I was younger, and it was another way of being weak. Whenever I would start to think that an opposing political party made a valid point, I would feel very guilty and feel like I need to change or fix it. It also probably didn't help that there was a ton of rhetoric flying around all the time that if you were part of an opposing party, there was something wrong with you. I internalized it all, which only fueled my fear of mistakes, but I have realized I am allowed, and should, come to my own conclusions about things.

All of this might not sound like OCD if you didn't know it, but my brain had convinced me that there was only one way to make sure I was me and not weak, only one way to live, and any deviation from that was met with panic, fear, guilt, and pain. But now I realize it is okay to be multi-faceted and in fact, it is good. I am still me when I do what I feel like rather than sticking to some rigorous rule that was arbitrarily and rigidly decided upon by my sticky brain.

# The Weight of the World

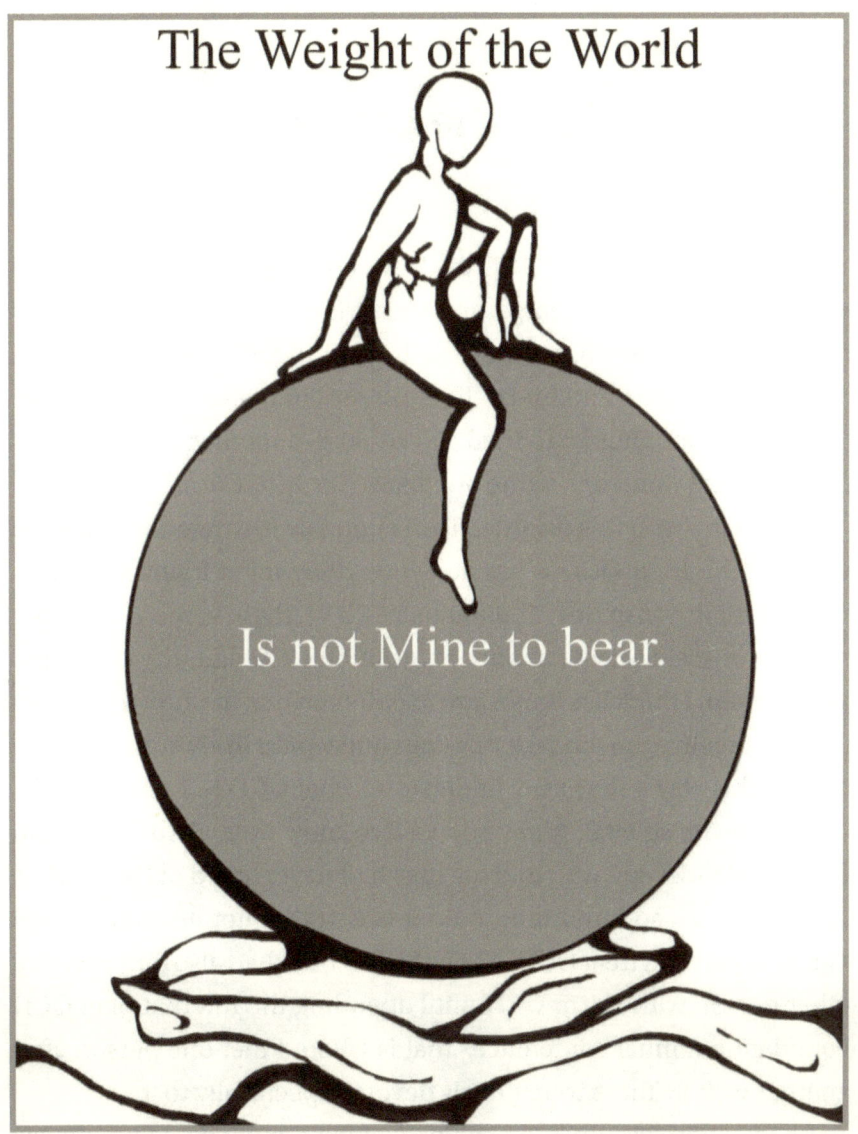

Is not Mine to bear.

**Illustration by Finn Conrey**

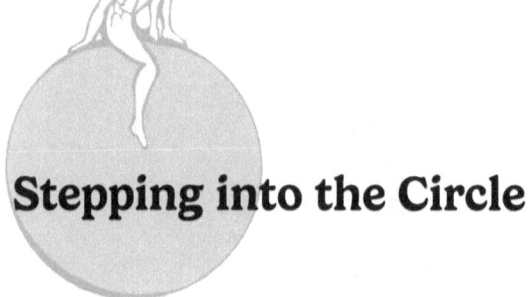

# CHAPTER 24

# Stepping into the Circle

The One Million Steps for OCD Walk was coming up, and I was excited to form a team with George and the girls to raise money for OCD research and outreach. I was eternally grateful for being able to go on the IOCDF website and find a therapist for Finn, one who helped her get her life back after I had tried all I could as a mother. I knew immediately what I wanted to name our team: *Not Your Cliché.*

Like many with this disorder, I am endlessly frustrated with people who use the term OCD as an adjective. They tell a friend who likes to keep their house tidy, "You are so OCD!" These same people put memes on social media about organization OCD, laundry OCD, and so on. Again, I think it is important to point out that many of these people don't realize the damage this does and would likely stop using the term in this way if they truly understood what OCD is. Education and awareness are so vital. Many counselors know little about OCD, and I've talked to several who told me they had never heard of Harm OCD. This is why it's so important to understand that not just any mental health expert can treat OCD. Not only that, but I had also only met one other person with Harm OCD until attending the International OCD Foundation annual conference. That is where I met one person after another with it. There were panels devoted specifically to it.

I have often felt if people could see how many people are deeply affected by this beast, they would understand that misusing the term OCD chips away at the serious consideration that should be given to those who are actually suffering from this disorder. When people who are struggling with it do ask for help or an hour or two off from work to go meet with a therapist, their boss may only have ridiculous memes running through his head or the image of an old roommate who claimed to be "So OCD" but only used the term with a snicker and a wink to get out of cleaning the toilet. Watering down this disorder is absolutely harmful to those who are suffering from the very real neurological disease that steals hours, days, and years from sufferers, and even takes lives. Our neurological disorder is Not Your Cliché. I thought it was the perfect team name.

We drove down to Newnan, Georgia, where the walk was to be held on a mild September morning. Katelyn, "Katie" O'Dunne, vice president of OCD Georgia, a lead advocate for the International OCD Foundation, and at the time, the chaplain at Woodward Academy in Atlanta greeted us. I learned she is a fellow runner, an ultra-marathoner—my kind of gal. She is a caring, welcoming soul who also knows the depth of struggle that OCD and particularly Harm OCD brings. More than that, she is willing to make herself vulnerable and share her story. She did exactly that a couple of weeks later at the IOCDF conference.

Before the walk began, I looked around at the people there. They were all ages and ethnicities. I knew from the fundraising page that many of them were clinicians, but many were people living with OCD as well. OCD has no preference for race or gender.

Katie instructed us to gather around and form a circle before we began the walk. "Thank you all for being here today. Before we start, I would like to take just a few minutes for anyone who might be willing to step into the circle and say a few words about why you are here. Share your journey, encouragement, or whatever you would like."

My heart was filled with so much gratitude for Finn's wonderful psychologist. Her patience, kindness, and wisdom. She wasn't at the gathering, but I wanted to say thank you in honor of her to the clinicians who were there. I highly doubted Finn would speak, and I had learned that in these situations, it was better for me to not push her to participate. However, I wanted to make sure my speaking would not make her so anxiety-ridden that she would be miserable.

I looked at her and mouthed. "Are you okay with me saying something?"

In reply she held up a finger for me to wait a minute.

I wasn't sure what that meant. I contented myself with listening to the stories of the other people who stepped into the circle one-by-one to share their experiences of bravely battling OCD, their journey with cognitive-behavioral therapy and exposure and response prevention therapy. They shared their gratitude for those who had helped them along the way: their families and therapists. I examined their faces and saw varying degrees of the battle-weary look I'd seen on Finn's face and my own. Some were downright haunted. Others seemed to have made it to the other side and bore the mien of hard-won post-battle confidence. They were living, breathing proof of freedom. Evidence that it could be done.

Then, to my complete shock, Finn raised her hand. Katie smiled at her and motioned for her to step into the circle.

## Finn Says:

I took a deep breath, raised my hand, ignored the little voices in the back of my head (something that I had only just recently figured out how to do) and I spoke. I talked about how I felt like people didn't understand OCD, and how I didn't want people to feel as alone or lost as I did. I spoke about different types of OCD, and how they are often overlooked.

And then I stepped back beside my mom. It wasn't anything major, but it felt like it to me. As someone who struggled for so long with anxiety and OCD, sharing my thoughts without feeling the need to do some sort of compulsion or clarification was so freeing. I didn't feel the eternal dread and terror in the back of my mind, nor did I overthink and pick apart every single thing I did. I simply said my peace and went back to my spot.

For most people, that was the norm. For me, this was a major accomplishment. I could do something without it all crashing down on my head in a fiery, spiraling inferno. That was not quite the first time I had seen the fruits of my labor, but it felt more satisfactory, seeing that I had made progress on the thing I had shown up there for.

After that, we went on the walk. We could leave whenever we wanted. I walked for a bit, and after a while, I told my mom that I was ready to go. That may not seem like much either, but before therapy I would have berated myself for not working harder, staying longer, walking farther, because I wasn't doing enough or wasn't fulfilling my OCD's and anxiety's expectations for myself. And yet, I said when I was ready to go and didn't beat myself up for it.

As I walked back to the car, I could joke around and talk with my family without over analyzing everything and worrying about every single reaction and how I need to fix things. I could even give my sister a piggyback ride. Before, when my OCD was more focused on her, I would have never been able to do that.

Now, none of this means I don't have OCD anymore. In fact, I will live with it for my whole life. But it doesn't control me like it used to. I can cope with it now and still live my life how I wish without being in constant panic and fear. I still mess up sometimes, and sometimes I have a bad day where my intrusive thoughts are louder than usual, but again, I can cope with it now, and I have the tools to live my life how I please.

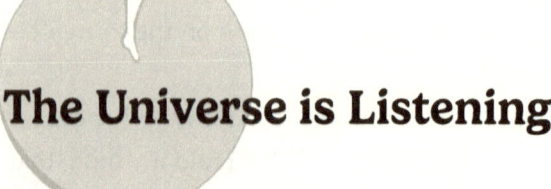

# CHAPTER 25

# The Universe is Listening

My daughter has come a long way from the dark days of lying on the floor sobbing while deep in the throes of OCD's demanding embrace, and so have I. At different times in our lives, we both managed to slip free from the bonds of scrupulous obedience, which promises assurance but delivers none. We've learned strategies, gained perspective, climbed the hill, and vowed to share that knowledge. So now that I have all this information and, at least to my thinking, moral responsibility to speak up, what will I do with it? When I'm confronted with misguided individuals using OCD to land a joke or sell a product, how will I respond? I should educate and inform. Spread the word, right?

Take it from me, the Universe is listening. No less than 24 hours after asking myself this grand question, I visit a street fair with my youngest daughter and look up to see a vendor with a giant banner that reads "OCD Fashions for You." Well, bless my crusading soul. I wanted to know what I'd do in such a situation, and the Universe said, "Wish granted. Have at it! Let's see what you do with this." The Universe snickered, grabbed a glass of lemonade—it was a hot July day in the Deep South and the Universe had sweat running down its back like an OCD sufferer filled with righteous indignation and ready to make a point—no wait, that was me. At any rate, the Universe sat back to watch me mumble and stumble my way through this lesson in practicing what I preach. After all, my last blogpost on harmocd-kimconrey.com had been about the annoyance of watching someone take a disorder that has stolen countless hours, years, and lives from its victims and reduce it to a cliché to market hand sanitizer. I'm ready. Nerves be damned. This is happening.

We know that declaration sounds brave in theory, but in practice it feels like a pounding heart, shaking hands, and a churning stomach. Ask anyone who has stood up for what they believe in, OCD or not. Most valiant moments start out with the hero about to vomit.

But then I notice . . . the vendor is a sweet-looking individual with an innocent smile.

"Hey, how's it going?" she asks.

"I'm good, thanks. These skirts are absolutely lovely. The colors are so vibrant." I feel oddly calm. I don't want to go to war with anyone. I'd rather simply connect. My youngest looks at the various patterns on the skirts while I have my moment.

"Thank you! I made all of them. Each one is unique."

"Well, they're fantastic."

"Thank you."

Even as I gear up to ask her what I really want to know, there are no nerves and no defensiveness. That all took flight once I realized something about her that is so easy to forget in a world where we seldom meet face-to-face anymore. She likely needs and wants the same thing most of us do: connection, understanding.

"What does the OCD stand for in the name of your business?"

"Oh, when I make these skirts, I have to have each one just right or it drives me absolutely crazy. I have to take them apart and redo them until they are right, but I feel like I can't stop making them either. So, I thought, why not just call it 'OCD Fashions for You'?"

Not a name I would have chosen, but this is a *dialogue* about mental health. Not an argument. Keep it *open*. "Okay, yeah, my daughter and I suffer from OCD, and I also write about it, and so your banner just caught my eye. Does it bother you, too, when people who don't have OCD or don't really understand what OCD is, use it to sell things, or like when someone says they have OCD just because they like things neat? They aren't panicking because it isn't neat. Yet they tell people, 'Oh, I'm *so* OCD' or 'You're *so* OCD.' Does that frustrate you?"

"Yeah, I doubt they're waking up in the middle of the night to fix something." I look into her eyes, searching for that same fright I've seen in the mirror after a night of checking the front door over and over again until I'm breaking out in a cold sweat as I did many years ago. I search them for the same helpless terror I detected in my daughter's eyes that brought me to my knees, begging God and the internet for help, combing the library shelves and insurance databases before finding the right therapist for her. Did I see this same horror in this woman's eyes? Truthfully, I'm not sure.

The lady really was a sweet soul, and we had a lovely conversation. I got a new skirt. Though I still don't know whether she has OCD, I'm not a health professional, and it isn't my place to judge. And yes, personally I would feel better if she would name her business something else. After all, I haven't heard of Cancer Creations or Parkinson's Pastries because that's wildly offensive, yet it's somehow okay to use OCD in this way. One thing I know for sure is that very few people ever change, for the better at least, with scorching accusations and ego-driven diatribes, but connection-driven dialogue from one human being to another can work wonders. Planting seeds that bloom later is a very real phenomenon.

And speaking for myself, I learned exactly what I would do when faced with a situation where I needed to stand up for what I believe in. I'm happy to report that the Universe is full of opportunities to grow and connect—to trade in ego for our better angels of understanding and compassion. I'm happy to say that when we think we are looking for confrontation, what we are often seeking is simply a connection. But I'm most happy to report that . . .

The Universe is listening.

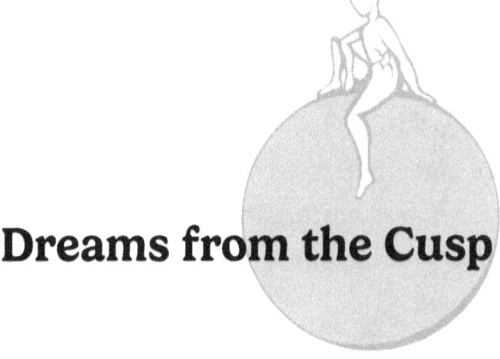

# CHAPTER 26

# Dreams from the Cusp

Finn and I sat on the couch having a conversation about girls, careers, and the future. Around this time, they also asked to begin being referred to with they/them pronouns. Now that the OCD was untangling itself from various thoughts and feelings, it was easier for them to get a clearer grasp on everything, really. Like who they truly are, and I was one proud mom to have a child with the courage to be exactly who they are.

Though OCD likes to vine itself into other experiences such that one needs surgical skills to dissect what is a normal worry and what is OCD, we were having more and more conversations that could be considered regular teenage worry about the future—and the present if they're looking to avoid homework.

"I think I finally understand what Dr. Yong meant by sitting with the discomfort of OCD."

I was overjoyed to hear this. Many tearful conversations had gone round and round with Finn telling me they didn't understand the concept of "sitting with" an uncomfortable thought. They feared it meant they agreed with the thought. "What finally worked for you?"

"Well, Dr. Yong had me read this book called *Needing to Know for Sure*.[12] There is an analogy in there about having an itch and refusing to scratch it. They said a thought is the same thing. It will itch for a while and be very hard to ignore, depending on how bad it itches, but if you do nothing, it will eventually stop itching. *That* I understand."

12    See endnote 7: Seif, Martin, PhD and Winston, Sally PsyD. (2019). *Needing to Know for Sure: A CBT Based Guide to Overcoming Compulsive Checking & Reassurance Seeking.* New Harbinger Publications.

"That's a perfect way to explain it. Yes!"

"Right?" They smiled.

We had come so far from the child I found lying on the floor sobbing and dry heaving. In fact, Dr. Yong even thought Finn was ready to move on from constant therapy. Which admittedly, scared the hell out of me.

I was having a nice, relaxing evening when Finn walked into the living room and said this: "Dr. Yong thinks I can discontinue therapy now."

If this were a cartoon, this would have been the point where steam shot out of my ears or my head exploded, but here in the real world I quietly panicked inside while trying to work out a non-confrontational answer that conveyed gentle concern without being a total nag and certainly without giving away the fact that I flat-out disagreed.

"So not even once a month?" I asked.

"Nope. I have it under control. We just don't have that much to talk about anymore."

But should I disagree? I trust her therapist. The woman is amazing! Also, I'm the mom, but *this isn't my therapy*. My child isn't even a minor anymore. I've also suffered with Harm OCD, and I know firsthand that it absolutely can reach a point where it no longer rules one's life. So why was I so scared?

*Stay with it. Breathe. What are you really feeling?*

The path to finding a good therapist was so long and fraught with false starts. For years, I felt alone as a parent struggling to help my child. I was barely hanging on, hoping they could just hold it together one more day, one more week, until the appointment with the next therapist. We went through so much before finally finding one with the expertise to deal with Harm OCD. When we finally found this godsend, this ERP (Exposure and Response Prevention)-certified, OCD-confronting angel from heaven with decades of experience in dragging that Harm OCD beast out into the light like a vampire screeching under the sun, I didn't want to let go. I wanted to hang on like the grim death that tormented the worst of my intrusive thoughts!

What if it returned?

What if Finn started melting down again and asking me if they deserved to live? As I thought back on those days, nausea hit me in waves.

The kneejerk answer to my questions might be, "You can't be pessimistic like that." But I didn't think I should be running from that possibility any more than an OCD sufferer should be running from an intrusive thought. What if it does recur?

Well, that's what this whole journey has been about, reaching the point where we take the training wheels off and they balance on their own.

I took a deep breath and said to them, "This is great! And if you ever need Dr. Yong in the future, you know where to find her."

They went on to tell me about a dream they'd had the night before. If the "subconscious is nature and nature never lies," as Carl Jung said, then perhaps Finn really was ready.

### *Finn says:*

In my dream, I was running around on an alien planet with a small crew of other people, and we were all trying to find a way out because whenever anyone tried to fly out on a ship they died. There was some sort of weird barrier around the planet. To make matters worse, we were each being chased by our own sort of alien or monster. The creature was specific to each person, and the fact that we were always running kept the crew from talking to each other for most of the time. The creatures would never tire, and they never stopped. Mine was a tall creature about 8 or 9 feet at least, and it was pitch black with white arms, hands, legs, feet, and its head was white. My creature had no other interest in any of the other crew and none of their creatures had any interest in me.

After a while, I noticed that the crew kept thinning out. I realized that either they had figured out a way off the planet or died trying. I saw no bodies, so I figured they must have been on their own ships. This was further reinforced when I ran to the ship dock and saw that some people's ships were gone. I did not have time to stay there and work it out, though—I had to keep running.

Like most people, I could not keep running forever, and it eventually caught up to me. When I stopped running, my creature stood a short distance away from me and just looked at me: not with anger, hatred, rage, or viciousness as I thought it would. It simply stood there with patience and some sort of care. As I thought about all our interactions, I realized it had never chased me as if it were hunting. It was simply quietly walking behind me, trying to catch up, only getting close when I would take brief pauses before running again. It did not speak in any words, but it slowly walked with me to my ship, helped me in, and showed me how to get off the planet without dying. I cannot remember what the trick was now that I am awake, but I remember that it waved as I left.

Later in my dream, I returned to the planet, but not to the present. I was there in the past like I was watching some sort of vision, and yet I had some slight control over what was happening. The world itself seemed more hostile, with cracks in the ground and plants far more overgrown than they should have been. I was there to observe the creature this time. I watched as some force magically pushed together several smaller creatures in the same space until they eventually fused into the one from my past, or rather, its future. This creature differed greatly from what it would eventually become—it was angry and lashing out at anything that came near it. It chased others around and seemed terrifying, but the more I watched it, the more I realized it was just confused, in pain, and lashing out because it was afraid. It was alone and didn't know who or what it was.

Eventually it spotted me and chased me, too. It had become what I feared, but it needed help. After running for a while, I reached a spot where it could see me but not reach me, and from there I tried to explain what was happening and how I was no threat. After a bit, everything seemed to click, and it calmed down, recognizing me as a friend rather than foe. Once it did, the world itself shifted, the landscape changed so that it could reach me. Not only that, but the surroundings became much less hostile and frightening. The cracks in the ground closed, and the plants shifted to a more reasonable size. We had come to some sort of understanding and felt care for each other. I remember little of what happened after that, other than some weird dream nonsense, but I remember it stayed by my side and tried to help.

When I looked back on the dream later, I think maybe the creature in the dream was me or part of me. I recently have been trying to rediscover who I am after years of burying it in order to fit this odd ideal that some part of me felt like I had to be. I ran from and denied the things that I loved and were a part of me for years because they did not fit the image of what I felt like I should be. I feel like that was the first part of my dream, where I was running from the creature. Lately, I have been trying to embrace the parts of me I felt like I could not before and have been much happier for it. That was the part of the dream where I finally let the creature catch up to me, and it treated me kindly.

In the flashback part of the dream, I think I was looking back on how, when I was younger, I had many fears about myself that stemmed from not only mental illness but also real and perceived pressures from society. I would, at times, lash out at people who I cared about, but I didn't know why. I was in pain, but I didn't know how to fix it or express it, so I just continued on as if everything was fine. The part of the dream where I convinced the creature that I was not a threat might have been more than one thing. When I was younger, I just wanted someone to say, "I am sorry you are going through this. I know you are exhausted. I am proud of you for making it this far; you are really doing your best," because I felt like I should always be trying harder. I was never doing enough. I was in pain because I was lazy; I thought, yeah, I am hurting, but I must be the cause somehow or this must be normal, and I am making a big deal out of nothing. I desperately wanted people to be patient with me and to understand I was really trying. I wanted my pain to be acknowledged. I wanted someone to offer a hand and meet me halfway. But I also felt like I didn't deserve it.

Me convincing the creature might have also been me comforting my younger self. Not only was the world hard on me, but *I* was hard on me. I still am hard on myself, but I am trying to do better, being gentle with myself rather than how harsh I had been in the past. I slip up sometimes, but I am trying to correct myself. Maybe I was also convincing myself that I am worth my love and care, and I am not the evil that I sometimes worry that I am. All the parts of me are worthy of love and attention no matter how strange they may seem, even to myself sometimes. After me and the creature reach an understanding, we become close. I think it was me learning to enjoy being with myself.

I found the dream to be a very eye-opening experience. It gave me a chance to learn to understand myself better. I hold the creature in high regard in my mind, to the point where a few days after my dream I drew the creature, so I knew it wouldn't be lost to time or the deepest corners of my mind.

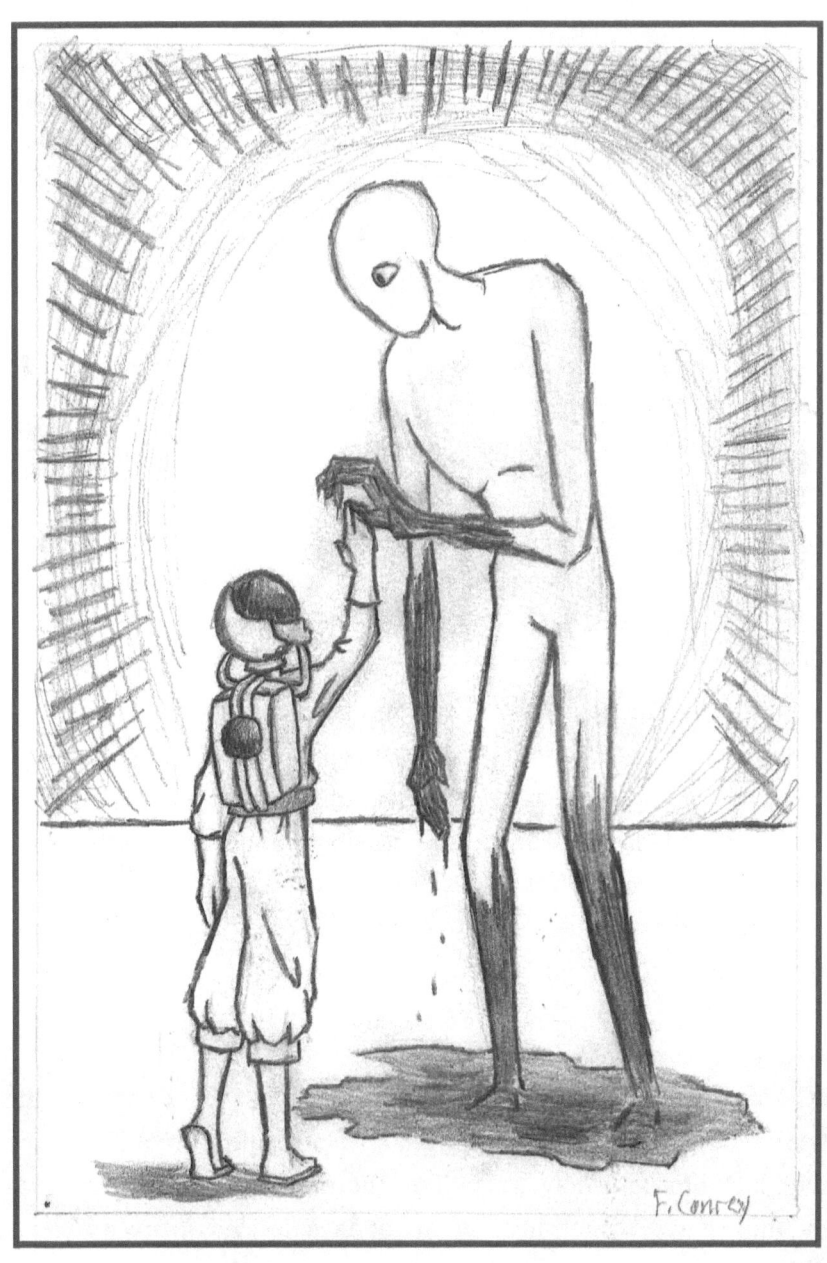

**Illustration by Finn Conrey**

I will say, though, the night after that I had a dream where I was in a life-or-death game with God to see who would survive the apocalypse. When the final dice rolled and landed, I heard a booming voice from the sky call down and say, "ONLY THE SEXY WILL SURVIVE." I scrambled, wondering if I would survive or not. So honestly maybe this is just an over analyzation of my dreams, but I learned some interesting things about myself.

After I finished laughing a little and telling Finn that I was sure thumping club music started playing after the dream deity's pronouncement that only the sexy would survive, I realized some truths about Finn's dream that applied to more than just them. As I thought about it, I couldn't help but see similarities in myself. They observed these fragments of themselves as they merged into one being, a being that wished to help them. I'd described myself as being fragmented, and the best I could do was pick up a fragment to offer to those I love.

Finn was on the cusp of being whole again, while I was recognizing my own tendency to be fragmented as well. At some point, we all have to stop running from those parts of ourselves that scare us and realize they are not foes at all but guides pointing the way to freedom.

There's a reason that a state of wellness is referred to as wholeness. Walking around in fragments is no way to live.

OCD is never cured. Decades after the emergence of it in my own life, it still creeps back, hoping to find a space to slither in: a little stress here, lack of sleep there. I'd written the number four, looked down, and there it was, something I might not have noticed on any other day, a four where the right angle didn't quite touch the line of the four. Who cares? Right? Well, no one should, and that's the point. But this is no ordinary four. Oh, no! That little tease is a gateway to misery. I want to close the four, take my pen and make one little mark, and I would, too, if I believed that would be the end of it, but it won't. I've been here before. This morning it will be that four, later that evening, I'll be checking a door that I already know is locked, or I'll be halfway out of my neighborhood before turning back around to check my garage door even though I know good and well it's closed.

It's not a number.

It's a trap.

I close the notebook and allow myself to acknowledge the discomfort, experience it. I remember a day when this would have felt impossibly hard, and I would have been sure something horrible would have occurred to someone I love if I walked away without closing the four.

I've come a very long way to make it to this point where I can walk away . . . and keep walking.

People with even severe OCD can get there, too.

Don't lose hope.

Going forward, we reclaim the strength in our vulnerability; the things that used to scare us become our guides. We've been here before: shaking, panicking, and cold sweating our way through the worst of it to come out on the other side with a stronger heart and gentler spirit. We take what we know from facing down these beasts that threaten our freedom and suck the joy from our life and share it with the next person we find barely making it through the night or combing blog posts day after day wondering if the intrusive images flashing through their minds make them a bad person or even a murderer.

I haven't found Finn on the floor crying and dry heaving over Harm OCD and its terrifying images in a long time. I hope never to again, but if I should, we know this beast—what feeds it, what starves it, and oddly, what gifts it leaves as it skulks away . . . compassion, knowledge, the ability to say, and mean it . . .

"You'll be okay."

# Epilogue

Three years later, I sit at my desk and type in my latest blog post at harmocdkimconrey.com. Sometimes OCD still gives me the stink eye, but these days I can wink, smile, and keep on walking. I know that millions still suffer, though. That's why I'm spreading the word about what OCD with intrusive thoughts is and how evidence-based treatment really can help.

Finn continues to do well. In fact, they're preparing for their biggest non-OCD-related challenge yet: to study abroad in Japan. Lord knows I'll miss Finn, but I'm excited for them. It's hard to imagine that a few short years ago, I was afraid they would lose their scholarship and leave their university due to OCD making their world smaller and smaller. Losing their scholarship had been the least of our worries. I'd been terrified Finn would lose their life! Now they're thriving. This is the power of good mental health services. If you need help, if your child needs help, don't be afraid to seek it out. Be tenacious. You're worth it.

Please join me in spreading the word about OCD and intrusive thoughts, and let's advocate together for good mental health. The International OCD Foundation has numerous resources to help you. Go to iocdf.org. Also, check out the National Alliance on Mental Illness. nami.org/Home

# REFERENCES

[1] Schwartz, Jeffrey, and Beyette, Beverly. (2016). *Brain Lock: Free Yourself from Obsessive-Compulsive Behavior: A Four-Step Self-Treatment Method to Change Your Brain Chemistry*. New York: Harper Perennial

Published over two decades ago, *Brain Lock* is a book that covers OCD in its many forms. It gives information for the curious mind about the causes of the disorder. It also covers treatment including medication and the authors "water wings" approach to meds, and his four-step approach to freeing oneself from the grips of OCD: relabeling, refocusing, and revaluing.

[2] Nicely, Shala and Hershfield, Jon. (2017). *Everyday Mindfulness for OCD: Tips, Tricks, and Skills for Living Joyfully*. New Harbinger Publications Inc.

This book is a must have for focusing on joy and compassion for self which can be sorely lacking in the person with OCD. It also teaches mindfulness, which is difficult for the OCD brain that tends to be stuck inside its own obsessions much of the time.

[3] International OCD Foundation. (2021). iocdf.org

This is an invaluable resource for those experiencing OCD and their caregivers as well. This site has the capability to search for therapists and support resources in your area. There is also fantastic information for loved ones trying to understand this disorder and treatment options as well.

[4] Hershfield, Jon. (2018). *Overcoming Harm OCD: Mindfulness and CBT Tools for Coping with Unwanted Violent Thoughts*. New Harbinger Publications Inc.

This book deals with Harm OCD specifically, and helps the reader understand what these thoughts are and what they are not—specifically that these thoughts are not indications that the person thinking them is a bad person. Hershfield demystifies the various treatment approaches, and helps the reader learn how and when to explain their disorder to loved ones.

[5] Apergis-Schoute, Annemieke. (2015). *Brain Scan Reveal Why it is so Difficult to Recover From OCD-and Hint at Ways Forward.* The Conversation. theconversation.com

This is a fascinating look at the OCD brain and its inability to decipher what is safe and what is not in a side-by-side comparison of a non OCD brain. This study gives insight into why it is so difficult for patients to understand that they are not in danger from a variety of compulsions: germs, intrusive thoughts, checking etc.

[6] Jansen, M., Overgaauw, S. & De Bruijn, E. (2020). *Social Cognition and Obsessive-Compulsive Disorder: A Review of Subdomains of Social Functioning. Frontiers in psychiatry*, 11, 118. doi.org

This study covers some interesting and understudied territory having to do with social cognition in those with OCD. There is some evidence that the OCD brain may have a difficult time processing social cues, especially those related to disgust. This is an excellent read for those that feel they have noticed a connection between their OCD and anxiety related to the emotions of others. This study also covers the effects of SSRIs on these findings.

[7] Seif, Martin, PhD and Winston, Sally PsyD. (2019). *Needing to Know for Sure: A CBT Based Guide to Overcoming Compulsive Checking & Reassurance Seeking.* New Harbinger Publications.

An excellent source for understanding and learning to break the loop of reassurance seeking OCD. It uses their Worried Voice, False Comfort, Wise Mind system to help the reader not only see themselves in the examples but also spot the traps that their OCD drags them into.

[8] Rasmussen, S.A., and M. T. Tsuang.. 1986. "Clinical Characteristics and Family History in DSM-III Obsessive Compulsive Disorder." American Journal of Psychiatry 143: 317-322. (Italicize American Journal of Psychiatry)

*Refers to statistics on back jacket copy of this book.

[9] Storch, E.A., C.W. Lack, LJ. Merlo, M.L. Jacob, and W.K. Goodman. 2007. "Clinical Features of Children and Adolescents with Obsessive Compulsive Disorder and Hoarding Symptoms." Comprehensive Psychiatry 48: 313-318. (Italicize Comprehensive Psychiatry)

*Refers to statistics on back jacket copy of this book.

# Acknowledgements

**KIM CONREY** wishes to thank Dr. Doug Smith, M.D., DLFAPA, for his expertise, encouragement, and humor. Thank you also to Dr. Martha Boone and Beverly Armento for their encouragement and endorsement. Thank you to the Roswell critique group, which has always made anything I've written better as they sat through many COVID-necessitated Zoom calls to listen and offer suggestions. The Wild Women Who Write have always been a sounding board and offered encouragement without fail. My heartfelt gratitude goes to Shala Nicely, LPC, for pointing this frazzled caregiver in the right direction and offering her kindness, direction, positivity, and light. Thank you to the International OCD Foundation for pointing the way for so many people for a while now. Thank you, Katie O'Dunne: she leads the way, consistently. Thanks go to my bestie, Cherie, for always listening: "Presence" is highly underrated. Finally, thank you to, Haley Swanson, author and former acquisitions editor at HarperCollins Wave for making me believe right from the start that this account "must be in the world." As always, thank you, George Weinstein, for your patience, kindness, and love on the writing journey and now, all our journeys together.

**FINN CONREY** would like to thank each and every family member for all their support, especially their wonderful mom who supported and empathized with them every step on this journey. They would like to thank their amazing therapist, who was so kind but also never put up with their crap. Finn would like to thank their best friend, Vincent, who was always willing to hear them out. Finally, they would like to thank every kind stranger and acquaintance who even offered the smallest passing word of kindness: they will probably never know each other and those individuals almost definitely will never know how those words helped give them confidence when they struggled with anxiety but Finn would like to thank them anyway.

## ABOUT THE AUTHORS

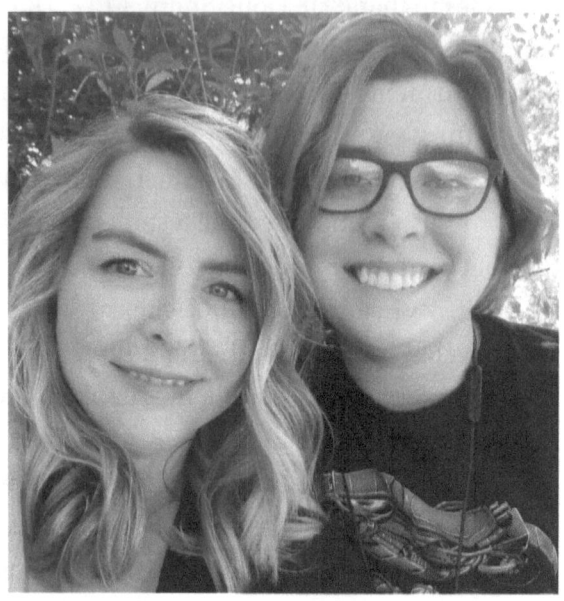

**KIM CONREY** is the Georgia Author of the Year recipient in the romance category. In addition to *You're Not a Murderer: You Just Have Harm OCD*, she's also the author of the sci-fi romance series Ares Ascending and the urban fantasy The Wayward Saviors series. She also serves as VP of Operations for the Atlanta Writers Club and podcasts with the Wild Women Who Write Take Flight. Head to harmocdkimconrey.com for more resources and blogposts about Harm OCD. To learn more about her fiction, head to kimconrey.com

**FINN CONREY** is an artist and writer constantly feeding their imagination to create illustrations and stories both fantastical and meaningful. They are currently making their way through life and all of its wonders with the loving support of their friends and family. Their work can be found at sloaneco23.wixsite.com/crypticmothcreations

# NOTE FROM THE AUTHORS

It is our sincerest hope that this book helped, educated, or inspired you in some way. Please leave a review on Amazon, Goodreads, Bookbub, or anywhere else so other readers may gain more insight. Please also feel free to get in touch at harmocdkimconrey.com.